The
Eye Exam

A Complete Guide

The Eye Exam
A Complete Guide

GARY S. SCHWARTZ, MD
ST. PAUL, MINNESOTA

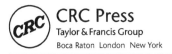

CRC Press
Taylor & Francis Group
Boca Raton London New York

CRC Press is an imprint of the
Taylor & Francis Group, an **informa** business

First published 2006 by SLACK Incorporated

Published 2024 by CRC Press
2385 NW Executive Center Drive, Suite 320, Boca Raton FL 33431

and by CRC Press
4 Park Square, Milton Park, Abingdon, Oxon, OX14 4RN

CRC Press is an imprint of Taylor & Francis Group, LLC

Schwartz, Gary S.
  The eye exam : a complete guide / Gary S. Schwartz.
    p. ; cm.
  Includes bibliographical references and index.
  ISBN-13: 9781556427558 (pbk. : alk. paper)
    1. Eye--Examinaion. 2. Eye--Diseases--Diagnosis.   I. Title.
  [DNLM: 1. Diagnostic Techniques, Ophthalmological--Handbooks.
  WW 39 S399e 2006]
  RE75.S34 2006
  617.7--dc22

                                         2005028744

ISBN: 9781556427558 (pbk)
ISBN: 9781003524137 (ebk)

DOI: 10.1201/9781003524137

DEDICATION

This book is dedicated to all those who have taken the time to teach me things over the years, be they parents, siblings, teachers, students, colleagues, patients, or friends—but especially to Suzanne.

CONTENTS

ACKNOWLEDGMENTS

I would like to acknowledge the assistance of those who helped this book make the journey from my head to your hands. First, thank you to Ed Holland—mentor, teacher, colleague, and friend—for showing me that it can be fun to write, teaching me the importance of wagon room, and allowing me to play Art Garfunkel to his Paul Simon. Also, thank you to Tim Olsen for taking time away from his family on a Saturday morning to teach me the proper way to do a fundus exam. It is amazing how one great teacher can reverse 10 years of entrenched bad habits in just a half an hour.

Thank you to Sanaz Afiat and Scott Sanderson for reading through the rough draft with an objective eye, and talking me into writing the chapter on motilities and alignment. Thank you to Lou Probst for recommending me for this project in the first place. Finally, thank you to John Bond, Amy McShane, Lauren Plummer, Monique McLaughlin, Megan Charlton, and everyone at SLACK Incorporated who first took a chance on me, and then put up with me.

ABOUT THE AUTHOR

Gary S. Schwartz, MD, is a comprehensive ophthalmologist in private practice in Saint Paul, Minnesota. He is an Adjunct Associate Professor in Ophthalmology at the University of Minnesota, where he teaches optics, refraction, and surgical techniques to ophthalmology residents and ophthalmic technologist students. He has received awards for his skills as a teacher from both medical students and ophthalmology residents at the University of Minnesota.

PREFACE

When I started out as an eye resident at the University of Minnesota in January of 1993, I was overwhelmed. I was struck by how poorly my training up to that point had prepared me for accomplishing anything very useful in the eye clinic. I searched for an all-inclusive, readable textbook that would tell me just what I needed to know to survive those first few months, without drowning me in detail. Needless to say, I didn't find anything that met with this description. So, I started to keep a little black notebook in my pocket.

When I heard something interesting, I wrote it down in this book. When I figured out a new way of thinking about an old problem, I wrote it down in this book. When I figured out an old way of thinking about a new problem, I wrote it down in this book. By the time I finished my residency in December, 1995, this little black book had a lot of things in it—some important and some trivial. As I leafed through it, I realized it represented a lot of the clinical theory I'd learned from my 3 years of working in the eye clinic. What it also represented was exactly the things I wished I'd known 3 years earlier when I was just getting started. I figured that there may very well be a few newcomers to the eye clinic (be they ophthalmology residents, optometry students, medical students, techs, assistants, or whoever) who, like I did way back when, wished they had a readable introduction to the eye clinic. I felt that my little black book, with some serious editing, could be expanded to become just that guide.

This book is meant to be an introductory guide to the eye clinic for the true novice. Its purpose is to teach you how to approach the eye patient, get a history, and properly use many of the instruments found in the eye clinic. Outside of refractive errors, this book is not meant to teach you about any eye diseases. However, by helping you be better at obtaining an eye history and physical examination, it should help you get a running start.

This book is organized in chapters and appendices. The first chapter should specifically help you learn to obtain a proper eye history, while subsequent chapters will help you in developing physical examination skills. The appendices are there for quick reference and will hopefully serve as a source for all those things that keep popping up that you just haven't memorized yet.

I hope you find this book useful.

Gary S. Schwartz, MD
St. Paul, Minnesota

Basic Basics

Welcome to the remarkable world of the eye clinic. It is certainly a wondrous place. There are a lot of patients, a lot of interesting pathology, a lot of treatment regimens, and a lot of people in white coats trying to piece it all together. There can be a lot going on, seemingly all at the same time, and if you're a novice, it can all look hopelessly confusing. Let's try to break everything down to the simplest elements. At its most basic, there are only 2 specific fundamental principles that help keep everything simple. They are as follows:

1. There are really only 3 complaints a patient can have:
   a. "My eye doesn't *look* right." It is red (injection), the lid droops (ptosis), the eye sticks out too far (proptosis), or one eye is always looking off in the wrong direction (strabismus), etc.
   b. "My eye doesn't *feel* right." It hurts (pain), bright light bothers it (photophobia), it feels like there's something in there (foreign body sensation), or it's itchy, etc.
   c. "My eye doesn't *see* right." Everything's blurry (decreased acuity), or double (diplopia), straight lines appear crooked (metamorphopsia), there are flashing lights (photopsias) or floaters (scotopsias), or areas of visual field loss (scotomas), etc.
2. If a patient has any pathology, you should almost always be able to actually see it and identify it in the clinic without having to do any invasive or expensive procedures.

As can be elucidated from the fundamental principles listed above, your approach to the eye patient needs to be broken down into 2 basic questions. Just about everything you do in managing each patient boils down to these 2 questions:

1. "What can or can't my patient see?"
2. "What can or can't I see in my patient?"

Table 1-1

ITEMS FOUND IN A STANDARD EYE HISTORY & PHYSICAL

HISTORY	*PHYSICAL EXAMINATION*
Identification	Visual acuities
Chief complaint	Manifest refraction
History of present illness	Motilities and Alignment
Past ocular history	Stereopsis
Past medical history	Pupils
Review of systems	Visual fields
Medications	Color vision
Eye Medications	External examination
Allergies	Anterior segment examination and gonioscopy
Family history	Intraocular pressures
Social history	Dilated posterior segment examination

You should be able to answer both questions almost every time with a good history (to answer, "what can or can't my patient see?") and physical examination (to answer, "what can or can't I see in my patient?"). There are a million and one different variations of the ophthalmic history and physical examination, but Table 1-1 provides a list of the fundamental items found in most complete eye exams.

It is important to understand the importance of writing a good history and physical exam. We are not just filling in blanks as part of an assignment that someone will be reading and grading us on (or worse yet, paying us based on). Rather, we are writing these for ourselves or our colleagues. We are recording as much useful information as we can to help us in deciphering our patients' current problems, thus letting us help cure them (which is why they come to us, after all). We are also writing things down that will help us when we see the patient the next time. This next visit may be 2 years later for a routine exam, 2 months later for a glaucoma patient, or 2 days later for an iritis or corneal ulcer patient. Regardless of how far down the road that next exam is, what we write down today will likely be the one clue we have in how that patient has progressed until we see him again. So, be careful what you choose to write down, and how you choose to do it.

THE HISTORY

Identification (ID)

This line is the one that states the patient's age, sex and race. Some may argue that putting the patient's race in this line is not relevant. However, pathology really can follow racial lines a lot of the time, and knowing a patient's race will often help in narrowing down a differential diagnosis. Examples of note include open angle glaucoma among African Americans, narrow angle glaucoma among Asians, and pseudoexfoliation glaucoma among Scandinavians.

Chief Complaint (CC)

The chief complaint is what brought the patient in to see you. Try to keep this simple. Record the patient's own words, but don't be afraid to use medical words where they are more descriptive. Examples include, "It feels like my glasses are foggy; I'm always trying to clean them, but it doesn't help," "My right eye drifts out," and frequently, "Straight lines look crooked." If you do use the patient's own words, surround the chief complaint with quotes.

History of Present Illness (HPI)

Some people also call the HPI the "History of the Chief Complaint" (HCC)—both terms get the same general idea across. The HPI is a systematic history of what has led up to the current problem. I find it best to start as far back in time as relevant and come forward to the present. Some clinicians prefer to start with the present and go back. Do whichever you choose, but try to be consistent.

If the patient complains of pain, you have to try to determine what type of pain he is experiencing. The general opinion is that there are only 2 types of pain that can be related to ocular pathology—*surface pain* and *ciliary spasm pain*. Surface pain is related to corneal irritation and tends to be expressed as feeling like there is something in the eye (between the eye and the lid). Surface pain tends to be very nonspecific—there are a lot of different actual problems with the cornea that can all present with the same type of pain. One important clinical tip is that surface pain will almost always go away if you put a drop of topical anesthetic into the patient's eye. If a patient has a sore eye, and it still hurts after placing a numbing drop, you need to look beyond the corneal surface to find the etiology of the discomfort.

Ciliary spasm pain is a deeper, more boring pain, and can signify that the patient is suffering from iritis. It tends to be associated with a brow headache, and is caused by spasm of the ciliary body. Ciliary spasm is also associated with *photophobia* (worsening of the discomfort with light), because light causes contraction of the iris, which pulls on the ciliary body, thus, exacerbating the ciliary spasm pain. Ciliary spasm is not relieved by topical anesthetics. It is, however, relieved with cycloplegics, which paralyze the spastic ciliary body, and act like placing a splint on a sprained ankle. Bear in mind that most patients with painful corneal pathology (eg, abrasion) will have ciliary spasm in addition to their surface pain, and thus may need cycloplegics for comfort even though the iris and ciliary body are not specifically involved with the injury.

Many patients will come to you complaining of itching/burning/foreign body sensation/pain. The best first question to ask these patients is, "What one symptom is the worst?" They will almost always be able to narrow it down to one symptom being worse than the others. Itching is generally representative of an allergic response, while burning and foreign body sensation point more toward blepharitis or dry eye. Another good question to ask is, "At what time of day are the symptoms the worst?" Blepharitis tends to be worse upon awakening, while symptoms of dry eye tend to get worse as the day goes on.

When a patient complains of any eye irritation or redness, it is imperative to get a contact lens history. Although contact lenses are generally safe and well-tolerated, at their most basic, they are bacteria-laden pieces of plastic sitting atop the cornea, and can be associated with their own specific collections of problems. First, ask if the patient wears contacts at all, and if he does, whether he wears soft, rigid gas permeable or hard ones. You need to establish wearing and cleaning habits and any recent changes in these habits. Importantly, you musk ask if the patient has recently slept in his contact lenses, which should immediately make you think of corneal ischemia and possibly a corneal ulcer.

Another question to ask is whether the patient has experienced this type of discomfort at any time in the past. If so, you will want to know if the symptoms follow any specific time course. Most allergy patients have worse symptoms in the spring, while most dry eye patients' symptoms are worse in the winter. You will also need to find out whether the symptoms always affect the same eye, or whether they can affect either or both. *Herpes simplex* virus keratitis and recurrent erosion are entities that can present with one eye being recurrently red and painful while the other eye remains asymptomatic.

Also, you should ask if the pain gets worse with eye movement. Most problems relating to the surface (corneal abrasion) or middle (iritis) of the eye won't be affected by eye movement. However, if the pain originates at the back (posterior scleritis) of the eye or the orbit (orbital myositis, optic neuritis), it will.

If the patient has any visual symptoms, it is very important to ask if the symptoms are monocular or binocular. Often, a patient will tell you that he is not sure, in which case you should tell him to cover each eye individually while sitting in your examination chair. You'll be amazed at how many patients complain of left eye blindness, for example, when in fact what they actually have is a binocular left visual field loss.

Diplopia, or double vision, is another complaint you will come across. Here, you must determine whether the 2 images are side-by-side (horizontal diplopia), one atop the other (vertical diplopia), or a combination. Try to elucidate whether the two images are the same clarity, or whether one is sharp while the other is blurry. You need to ask whether the diplopia occurs with one eye or both eyes open. *Monocular diplopia*, double vision with one eye open, is usually caused by the splitting of light from a corneal abnormality or cataract. *Binocular diplopia*, double vision with both eyes open, is usually from a strabismus (the 2 eyes are looking in different directions). Finally, you need to find out if a patient's double vision is worse when he looks in a particular direction, as this will help you isolate a weak or restricted muscle. Don't be fooled into assuming that the problem is a near vision one if the patient complains that he has diplopia when reading up close, but it goes away when he looks far away. It may be that the diplopia is brought out when the patient looks down, and he only notices it when he looks down to read.

If a patient complains of blurriness in vision, you should ask him to try to better explain the symptoms, and thus help you pinpoint the source of the problem. If he tells you that things just look "blurry," or "cloudy," "fuzzy," or something similar, the problem is probably very far anterior. These types of symptoms may be from the cornea (edema, epitheliopathy, scar), or can be from the lens (cataract). If the problem is located in the retina, the abnormal vision will usually be described as a *metamorphopsia* rather than blurriness. A patient is describing metamorphopsia when he tells you that straight lines appear wavy or crooked, or that the image seen with one eye appears smaller or larger than the image seen with the other. If a patient has these types of complaints, you should look to the retina for the source.

You should also ask if any specific episode led to the current complaints. Be careful not to get fooled here. In many cases it is straightforward: "A bug flew into my eye, and since then it has been red and sore." Some, however, are not straightforward, and may even be misleading. Occasionally, you may see a man, for instance, with a hand motion cataract, one that has developed slowly over decades, who is convinced that his monocular blindness is related to the fact that he hit his head getting out of the car the day before. What has happened here is that after hitting his head, he covered each eye with his hand as a quick check to make sure everything was working correctly. When he covered his good eye, leaving his hand-motion eye uncovered, he suddenly noticed he couldn't see out of it, thus making his 20-year cataract seem like an acute event.

Past Ocular History (POHx)

Here, you record any previous eye pathology or eye surgery your patient had prior to seeing you. You should also record spectacle and contact lens history here. Remember with contact lenses, you need to know the type of lens, how often they are replaced, type of cleaning regimen and any recent changes in wearing habits. It is imperative to find out how often your patient sleeps in their lenses. Don't forget to ask if the patient had ever had a lazy eye or ever had to have 1 eye patched as a child. Eliciting this history may give a clue to a history of amblyopia in a patient where one eye's visual acuity is less than predicted by the physical examination.

Previous eye surgery is an important part of the history to obtain. Patients with prior retina surgery, for instance, will have different problems, presentations, and needs than those with prior glaucoma surgery. Also, patients with a prior glaucoma or retina laser procedure will be different than patients with prior glaucoma or retinal open surgery. If a patient can't recall exactly what they had, you can often tell by examining them quickly with the slit lamp.

Past Medical History (PMHx)

Here is where you write down all medical problems that your patient has experienced to date (excluding all the specifically eye-related things). Most of the surgical things will truly be things in their past, and should be recorded as such. Examples include history of appendectomy, hysterectomy, or broken arm repair. Most of the medical histories will be ongoing, but are still part of the *past* medical history. These may include diabetes mellitus, asthma, or high blood pressure. For diabetes, you should always record the number of years that the patient has had it, as this has direct relevance to the health of the eyes.

Review of Systems (ROS)

The review of systems is where you record how a patient has been feeling lately. This represents the current overall health of the patient, and should not just be a rewriting of everything in the PMHx, unless there is something new. So, although "diabetes mellitus" would be something that is written in the PMHx, you would record "recent hyperglycemic episodes" under the ROS. A review of systems is just that, a review of the patient's organ systems. A typical list will include a review of the following organ systems: constitutional, respiratory, gastrointestinal, cardiac, musculoskeletal, endocrine, neurological, genitourinary, skin, ENT, and others. Many eye exam forms will have these listed out to help you remember them.

Medications

List what medications a patient is taking. To be complete, you need to write the name of the medication, the dosage, and how many times a day it is taken. A lot of older patients who take a lot of medications and see a lot of doctors will often have written this all out on a sheet of paper they carry with them. Many will often have a photocopied copy ready for you.

Eye Medications

When you ask a patient what medications he takes, don't forget to specifically ask drops what eye drops he takes. Even in the eye clinic, many patients may forget to include eye drops when listing medications. Be sure to specifically ask what over-the-counter medications he has been taking, as well. Knowing that a red-eye patient has recently been using over-the-counter vasoconstrictors or preserved lubricants may help you narrow down your differential diagnosis and establish your treatment options. Don't forget to ask what oral over-the-counter medications your patient is taking. These may include anti-inflammatories and allergy medications.

Allergies

Record what medications the patient is allergic to, and what the reaction was for each one (eg, rash, difficulty breathing, nausea). Be sure to include reactions to systemic medications as well as eye drops. By convention, data for this section should be written in red.

Bear in mind that when patients react to eye drops, they are often reacting to the preservative in that particular drop, rather than the active medication. Therefore, a different medication with the same preservative may lead to the same reaction. Conversely, the same medication with a different preservative may not lead to any reaction at all.

Family History (FHx)

The family history takes into consideration medical diseases as well as eye diseases. You often will get "no" for an answer if you ask "Are there any eye diseases in your family?" You'll get better results if you ask more specifically, such as, "Does anyone in your family see poorly?", "Is there anyone in your family who sees so poorly that he doesn't drive a car?", "Does anyone in your family have night blindness or color blindness or glaucoma?", and the common, "Did anyone in your family have a lazy eye or ever have to wear a patch over one eye as a child?" Do not forget to include all medical diseases in the patient's family (eg, heart disease, cancers).

Social History (SoHx)

Here, you want to find out about the patient's vocation and avocations. These are especially important when treating presbyopes with readers or bifocals. What they do at work (airline pilot, carpenter, computer operator) and in their free time (piano, needlepoint) will determine the strength, and often shape and location, of the bifocal add. This will also help you to know whether or not to recommend safety glasses.

Under social history, you also need to determine the patient's alcohol and tobacco history. You should also determine his living situation and (especially in older patients) the level of independence.

That completes the history part of the tour and takes us to the physical examination.

THE PHYSICAL EXAMINATION

Visual Acuities

Visual acuities are explained in detail in the next chapter. Basically, you want to establish what the patient's visual acuity is three different ways. You need to know the acuity:

1. At distance (20 feet) with their current glasses on
2. At distance (20 feet) through a pinhole
3. At near (14 inches) with their current glasses on

Be sure that you measure one eye at a time and that the occluded eye is really occluded (especially in children). The theory behind the pinhole is discussed in Chapter 3, but basically, the pinhole gives you an idea of what the patient's best corrected visual acuity should be.

Refraction

Refraction, the cornerstone of what we do, is discussed in detail in Chapters 4 through 6. Manifest refraction (MR) is done without drops, and necessitates the examiner being alert that the patient is not accommodating during the evaluation. Cycloplegic refraction (CR), on the other hand, is done while the patient is cyclopleged with eye drops (usually atropine or cyclogyl). Cycloplegia paralyzes the patient's ability to accommodate and thus gives you an idea of what his true baseline refractive state is without any accommodation. As you will learn in Chapter 6, accommodation adds plus power to a patient's refractive state by fattening and shifting forward the crystalline lens of his eye. Accommodation makes far-sighted people less far-sighted, normal people near-sighted (allowing them to see at near which is, of course the purpose of accommodation in the first place), and near-sighted people more near-sighted. The CR is most useful in young children who have such strong abilities to accommodate, that an MR may not give you much useful information.

Motilities and Alignment

This is discussed in detail in Chapter 7.

Stereopsis

Stereopsis is your brain's ability to fuse the 2 slightly different images seen by the 2 eyes into a single, three-dimensional (3-D) picture. Stereopsis is what makes 3-D movies and pictures so interesting to look at. When we measure stereopsis, we can get information about how well a patient is able to use both eyes together. For this reason, it is a great test to pick up subtle amblyopias (lazy eye) or strabismus (wandering eye) that may otherwise get missed. The amount of stereopsis that a patient can appreciate is measured in "seconds of arc"—the lower the number, the better the result.

In order to test for stereopsis, you must present a different image to the left eye than you do the right one. Special filtered pictures are used for this, and the patient must wear special glasses to view them properly. These glasses use polarized lenses to ensure that your patient's right eye is presented with something different than the left one.

There are many different versions of the stereopsis pictures that your office may have. The easiest one to see is the stereo fly. Here, the patient merely has to identify whether he appreciates that the wings of a fly appear to be elevated out of the plane of the picture. A positive test means that the patient has at least 200 seconds of arc of stereopsis, which isn't much.

A better way to quantitate stereopsis is via titmus animals (children) or circles (adults). Here the patient is presented with a series of pictures with decreasing seconds of arc of separation. The patient is first shown the easiest one and asked if he can see which part of the picture appears suspended above the plane of the rest. If he gets it correct, he is presented with the next most difficult picture and so on. These tests can usually measure someone's stereopsis down to 40 seconds of arc.

Pupils

You can glean a lot of information from a good pupil exam. For every pupil, you need to describe the shape, size in the dark, size in the light, and speed with which it changes size. You also need to compare each pupil to its partner, and determine if any anisocoria or relative afferent pupillary defect (RAPD or Marcus-Gunn pupil) is present. Some general doctors and nurses may use the abbreviation of PERRLA ("pupils equal and round, reactive to light and accommodation"). Although this may be adequate for their needs, it does not convey enough information to find a place in the eye clinic note.

In describing shape, bear in mind that normal pupils are essentially round. Previous surgery or trauma can make a pupil unround. Sometimes, this unroundness is caused by a break in the iris sphincter muscle at the pupillary border. These sphincter tears can almost always be seen by slit lamp biomicroscopy. At other times, the iris may be either caught in a surgical wound or pulled by some element of pathology such as a haptic of an intraocular lens or a strand of vitreous. In these cases, the pupil tends to be peaked in one sector giving it a teardrop shape, instead of the normal, round one. The peak of the pupil almost invariably "points to the problem," thus, giving you a clue as to where to look.

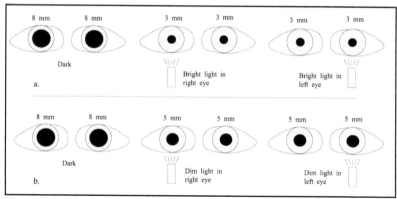

Figure 1-1. a. Both eyes constrict briskly and equally when a bright light is shone into either one. b. Both eyes constrict less briskly, but still equally, when a dim light is shown into either one.

A congenital deformity can also leave a patient with an unround pupil, so sometimes it is helpful to ask for old photographs for comparison. Patients with blue eyes will often be able to give a better history for an abnormal pupil than those with brown eyes, because the pupils of blue-eyed patients are so much more noticeable. Inflammation, with posterior synechiae (where the iris sticks to the lens positioned just behind it) is something else that can lead to an unroundness of the pupil.

An important piece of information to gather is whether or not a patient has a _relative afferent pupillary defect_ (RAPD). The RAPD is a "defect" because the 2 eyes do not work symmetrically because one is _defective_. Second, it is "pupillary" because, although the etiology of the pathology does not lie within the pupils themselves, it is picked up by examining the _pupils_. Third, it is "afferent" because the problem lies in the pathways that bring information _to_ the brain _from_ the eyes. Fourth, it is "relative" because either eye tested alone may appear normal, and the defect is seen only when the response of one eye is _compared_ to the response of the other.

Although RAPD is an afferent thing, it relies on the idea that the efferent pathways to the pupils are completely crossed. Thus, the brain cannot tell one pupil to constrict or dilate without telling the other to do exactly the same thing (Figure 1–1). However, at the level of the optic nerves, anterior to the optic chiasm, the afferent pathways are completely uncrossed. That is, all the information from the right eye is in the right optic nerve, and all the information from the left eye is in the left optic nerve.

The pupillary light response, at its most basic, is quite simple: if you shine a light into a patient's eyes, his pupils constrict. We can, however, break this down further to help understand the RAPD response:

1. If you shine a _bright_ light into a patient's 2 eyes, both pupils constrict quickly and fully.

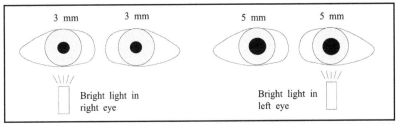

Figure 1-2. If a patient has an optic nerve problem affecting the left eye, it is possible that the pupils will constrict less fully when a bright light is shone into the left eye than when the same light is shone into the right eye. When comparing the response of the left eye to that of the right eye, it can be seen that this patient has a relative afferent pupillary defect.

2. If you shine a *bright* light into a patient's right eye only, both pupils constrict quickly and fully.
3. If you shine a *less-bright* light into a patient's right eye only, both pupils constrict less-quickly and less-fully.

Let's say that the patient has a problem with his left optic nerve (eg, optic atrophy, late stage glaucoma, or optic neuritis), and the right one is totally normal (Figure 1-2). What happens as we swing a flashlight from one eye to the other and back again? When we shine the bright light into his right eye, it is perceived as a bright light, and both eyes constrict quickly and fully. However, when we move that same light over to his left eye, because of his left optic nerve problem, the light is perceived as less-bright. Both pupils constrict less-quickly and less-fully than when the light is shone into the right eye. Because both pupils had been fully constricted when the light was shone into the right eye, they will *dilate* some when the light is moved to the left eye. Both pupils then *constrict* again when the light is moved back to the right eye. Remember that the right pupil and left pupil are always dilated the same amount in relationship to each other. We are not measuring an anisocoria (an *efferent* problem); we are measuring RAPD (an *afferent* problem).

RAPD can be measured even if the eye that you are interested in has a pupil that does not change size. The best example of this is someone who has sustained significant trauma, and has a permanently dilated pupil and possible traumatic optic neuritis. It would be nice to be able to look for an RAPD to evaluate the traumatic optic neuritis, even though that pupil does not move. We can do the whole RAPD exam while looking at the *other* pupil—the one from the uninjured eye. Let's say the left eye is the injured one. We look at the right pupil while we shine a light into the right eye. It constricts to 3 mm. We swing the light to the injured left eye, but still look at the right pupil. Now the right pupil dilates up to 6 mm. We shine the light back into the right eye, and it shrinks to 3 mm again. We have just diagnosed

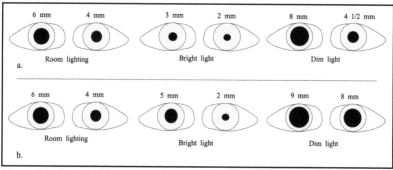

Figure 1-3. Patient (a) has anisocoria secondary to a sympathetic defect in the left eye. Note that the anisocoria is worst in dim light because the left eye has difficulty dilating. Patient (b) has anisocoria secondary to a parasympathetic defect in the right eye. Note that the anisocoria is worst in bright light because the right eye has difficulty constricting. It is important to understand that these two patients look exactly the same in normal room lighting, and that the nature of the anisocoria is not made evident until the lights are brightened and dimmed.

the left eye as having an RAPD without ever actually looking at it. This technique is called the *reverse RAPD* technique.

Another modification on the RAPD test is the *subjective RAPD* test. This test is done by merely asking a patient which eye the light looks brightest while looking for an RAPD. If a patient has a mild RAPD, and you're not really sure if you're seeing one or not, it may be helpful to ask, "Does the light look brighter in one eye than the other?" If the patient says, "Yes, it looks about half as bright in the left eye as the right," that means that he probably does have a real RAPD there. The subjective RAPD test is not a strong enough test to stand on its own, but it can be a helpful adjunct to the standard RAPD test.

Anisocoria, as we have said, is an efferent problem where, for some reason, the 2 pupils are different sizes in respect to one another (Figure 1-3). For the sake of this discussion, let's disregard non-neurologic causes of pupillary abnormalities (eg, sphincter tears, surgical or traumatic iris injuries). If one pupil is too big, it is not constricting enough, and the anisocoria is usually secondary to a problem with the sympathetic innervation that comes from cranial nerve III. If one pupil is too small, it is not dilating enough, and the anisocoria is usually a problem with the parasympathetics. The tricky part is to figure out if one pupil is too big or if the other one is too small. The easiest way to figure this out is to look at the pupils in light and dark. If the anisocoria is worse in the light, then the pathology must lie with the larger pupil which isn't constricting well, and the problem probably lies with the parasympathetics. If the anisocoria is worse in the dark, then the pathology must lie with the smaller pupil not dilating properly, and the problem can usually be found with the sympathetic system.

Visual Fields

Formal visual field testing (eg, Humphrey, Goldmann) is obviously not done on every patient who comes into your examination lane. This overuse of technology would be unnecessary as well as impractical. However, confrontation visual fields (CVF) are easy enough to perform in your lane and can give you enough information that it should be performed during every complete eye examination. Cover one eye of your patient well and have him look at your nose with the other one. Then test his peripheral vision in the other eye by asking the patient to count your fingers, or tell you when he sees your fingers wiggling, as you move your hand from his peripheral toward his central vision. Do not forget to test the central vision looking for central scotomas. You should repeat this while having him appreciate colors in all areas of the visual field. The easiest way to do this is to ask him to observe the color of the red cap of an eye drop bottle as you move it into all fields. Patients with subtle visual field deficiencies may be able to count fingers well in certain areas, but may see the red cap as black or gray in those same areas. Then repeat the test on the other eye.

You then need to better evaluate the central visual fields. The best way to do this is with an Amsler grid, which is a grid made up of small squares. Each small square is 5 mm-by-5 mm and subtends 1 degree when held at 30 cm from the eye. The whole grid, then, takes up the central 20 degrees of a patient's visual field. To use the Amsler grid correctly, have a patient cover one eye. While he has his reading glasses on, and *is staring at the dot in the middle of the grid*, ask:

1. Do you see the dot in the middle?
2. Do you see all four corners?
3. Are the lines of the grid straight, or are they wavy?
4. Are there any areas where the grid is missing or faint?

Document any unusual answers. I've found that the best way to document Amsler grid abnormalities is to draw exactly what the patient describes. Remember, that as with all types of visual field recording, you record the Amsler grid in the same orientation as it looks *to the patient*. Thus, left on your paper corresponds to left on the patient's visual field, and right on your paper corresponds to right on your patient's visual field. This orientation is in direct contradistinction to the rest of your physical exam where you record things as they look to you while you look at your patient in your examination chair. Your patient's left retina, then, is always drawn on the right side of the page because when you look at your patient, his left eye is on the same side as your right hand.

Color Vision

About 8% of males and 1% of females are born with an abnormality in their perception of color. For these patients, it is important to document that they have a deficiency. However, it is more important to find a new color deficiency in someone who had previously been documented as having normal color vision. In these cases, color blindness may represent a problem with the retina (toxic maculopathy) or optic nerve (optic neuritis). For this reason, color vision should be tested during every routine follow-up visit. Also, the color vision tests should be performed on each eye separately; it is not a binocular test.

There are many methods to evaluate a patient's color vision. Many of them, such as the Farnsworth D-15, and Farnsworth-Munsell D-100 are time consuming, technically difficult to administer, and require special lighting. These should be reserved for patients with specific eye problems, and are not part of the routine examination.

The best way to measure color vision as part of the routine examination is via the isochromatic color plates. The most commonly used of these are the Ishihara color plates. This test consists of a series of numbers made up of colored dots, placed against a background of different colored dots. Each plate has one number on it. A patient with a certain color deficiency will have trouble recognizing the number from the background on one or more than one of the plates.

To administer the Ishihara isochromatic color plate test, merely have a patient cover one eye and show him the plates one by one. Ask him what number he sees on the plate, and keep track of how many the patient gets correct. Then, merely record the number of correct plates over the total number of plates you presented for each eye. For example, if he recognized 10 plates correctly with the right eye, and 11 plates with the left, and you showed 14 plates, you will record it "OD: 10/14; OS: 11/14."

External Examination

The external examination is often forgotten because it doesn't entail the use of any special equipment or machinery. To perform a good external exam, look at your patient while you are talking to him and observe the lids, brows, blink rate, and so on. You can manipulate the lids a little bit if you need to. The external exam is where you can best evaluate ptosis, dermatochalasis, brow ptosis, and other problems of the ocular adnexa.

Anterior Segment Examination and Gonioscopy

This is discussed in detail in Chapters 8 and 9.

Intraocular Pressures

This is discussed in detail in chapter 10.

Dilated Posterior Segment Examination

This is discussed in detail in Chapter 11.

2

Examining Children

When dealing with small children, you really only need to do 2 things differently than you do with your typical eye exam. First, make the child comfortable. Second, adjust your exam technique accordingly.

MAKING THE CHILD COMFORTABLE

You should do whatever is in your power to make the child's experience as positive as possible. Remember that most trips to doctors' offices have some degree of unpleasantness attached to them. With all the vaccinations that children receive nowadays, it seems that every time that they are in a doctor's office they are getting an injection. It's helpful to distance yourself from the shot-giving clinics the best you can. If the child is old enough to understand and appears nervous, it is OK to come right out and say, "don't worry, we are not the types of doctors who give shots."

If your clinic is the type where everyone wears white coats, it may be helpful if you take it off when you're seeing children. Children will know you are a doctor, nurse, or technician if you're wearing a white coat, and will associate you with the people who are giving them injections. If you don't have a coat on, they may not know what to make of you straightaway, and give you the opportunity to form a relationship without their being too afraid.

If you see a fair number of children, try to set up a separate children's play area filled with safe toys, books, and maybe even a DVD player or VCR playing children's movies. The children will enjoy their visit more if they have something to do while waiting to see you. Their parents will enjoy the fact that their kids are being entertained, and the other patients will enjoy the fact that these children are being entertained in a separate area, leaving the remainder of the lobby quieter.

It is important for the child to understand that they are the patient and, therefore, the focus of your attention. For any child older than 3 or 4 years of age, I walk into the exam room, ignore the parents, and immediately start talking to the child. I extend my hand to the child, and say something like, "Hello, I'm Dr. Schwartz. How are you today?" This sends the message to the child that they are the most important person in the exam room. After examining the child, I then explain what I found to the child. The parents will be in the room to hear it, but I typically don't tell it directly to them. I have found that children appreciate it when an adult takes the time and energy to talk directly to them. I've also found that parents don't feel left on the sidelines with this approach—they appreciate it too.

It is nice to have a lot of small and colorful toys handy when examining children. Toys serve a lot of different purposes in the eye clinic. First, they show the child that you can be fun, and, therefore, are not someone to be feared. More importantly, however, they trick the child into looking at things. A child may not be as responsive as an adult to commands such as "look to the right" or "look at my ear." However, if you pick up a colorful toy and move it to the patient's right, he will usually look at it, and thus look to the right. One general rule here is "one-toy-one-look." This means that children will usually get bored with looking at a specific toy after a short period of time, and therefore you should have a pocket or drawer full of different toys if you are going to be doing exams on children.

Try to have some small token to give to the child as a reward. Most kids like stickers, and most clinics will have rolls of these for this purpose. Some kids look at the sticker as a reward for being brave and helpful. Others look at it as a payment for putting up with such unpleasantries.

If a child is a repeat client to your clinic (eg, for monthly amblyopia checks), try to ensure that he sees the same people every time. This will make the clinic look a lot less big and scary. Go out of your way to try to have the same technician or assistant check him in every time. A lot of children will bond to that one tech, and may be surprised if they come to a doctor's appointment and their doctor is there, but their special tech is home sick.

Try to make sure that the person doing the most important part of the exam is not the person giving the drops. Receiving eye drops is the most traumatic part of the exam for small children, and they may hold a grudge against anyone who does this to them. If you are the person who will be doing the cycloplegic refraction or the fundus exam, you should let someone else do the drops. Just walk out of the room saying something like, "Andy will be back in a minute to help out." Then let Andy come in and give the drops. By not telling the child what Andy was going to be doing, you make it look like it was Andy's idea, and you are off the hook. The patient still has trust in you, and should let you do what you need to. Andy may be out of favor with that particular patient, but because he doesn't have to do anything too important to that patient that day, it really doesn't matter in terms of getting a good exam.

Remember that children do get tired out during the exam, especially if they do a lot of crying. As they get tired, they tend to get irritable, and your ability to examine them will likely diminish. Don't be afraid to send the child home without the examination being completely finished, and have them come back on another day when you are both fresh. If you have not done the cycloplegic refraction yet, give the parents a prescription for atropine and have them give it to the child a couple of times over the 12 to 18 hours before the exam. This will ensure good dilation, while also ensuring that no one in your clinic is viewed as the bad guy.

You should always have the parent in the exam room if at all possible. The exam is a much less scary experience if their parent is in the room with them. I'll usually let the real little ones sit on the parent's lap on the exam chair. Remember that these chairs are built for adult-sized people, and the parent's lap can act as a kind of warm, cozy, and familiar booster seat. Also, you can use the parent to help hold the child if necessary. If the child is sitting on the parent's lap, he can easily hold the child's hands down or head still during the exam.

There is a less traumatic way to lie a young child down for a difficult exam if both parents are there (if only one parent is there, it works with a parent and a tech/nurse). One parent should sit on the exam chair. The other parent should sit on another chair so the two parents are facing each other and their knees are touching. Lie the child back so the head is on the lap of one parent, and the feet are on the lap of the other. One parent gets a good hold of the head and arms (to stop any potential flailing), while the other gets a good hold of the feet and legs (to stop any kicking). The doctor can then have both hands free to get a good look at the eyes. I've found this to be the least traumatic way to safely examine an otherwise frightened patient.

ADJUSTING THE EXAMINATION

When evaluating anyone's visual acuity, it is important to remember that you are always measuring things one eye at a time. It should be common sense that when you are measuring the visual acuity of the right eye, the left eye is occluded. With adults, this is easy. Just give them an occluder and say, "Please cover your left eye." With children, this is not so simple. For one thing, kids tend to squirm, and the occluder may shift out from in front of the eye that it is supposed to be occluding. Also, kids don't understand the purpose of the test. You are checking their vision to get an objective measurement of their visual function, but they think you are testing them, and that they could get punished if they get some of the answers wrong. For that reason, if they have one good eye and one bad one, they may actually cheat a little and uncover the good one a bit when you're trying to evaluate the bad one. They may not even do it intentionally. For that reason, you have to stay on top of things and constantly observe younger patients. If they are cheating by looking around the occluder, or just can't get the hang of holding it, you are better off by just taping an adhesive occluder over their eye and proceeding that way.

Measuring Visual Acuity

You should always measure a child's visual acuity with the most sophisticated system that he can tolerate. The gold standard for measuring someone's visual acuity is the Snellen eye chart, a chart made up of lines of letters of increasingly larger size. However, it is dependent upon a child's being able to recognize all of their letters. Most children can't handle this task until they're grade-school age—5 or 6 years old, so different ways of checking visual acuity had to be developed for those under age 5.

If a child cannot handle all the variety of a Snellen chart, he may do well on an "H-O-T-V" chart. This chart is similar to the Snellen chart, but it is only made up of the letters "H", "O", "T", and "V." This is a good selection of letters because it tests a child's ability to see horizontal shapes, vertical shapes, slanted shapes, and round shapes. Also, all of the letters are symmetrical (the left half is a mirror image of the right half). So if the child has the habit of drawing certain letters backward, this shouldn't pose a problem with this test. What is perhaps nicest about the "H-O-T-V" test is that shy children don't have to say anything during the exam. You can give the child a sheet with the 4 letters written on it to hold on their lap. If you point to a letter on the screen, the child only has to point to the letter on the sheet on their lap. Another advantage is that you can send the parent home with a copy of this sheet so their child can practice up at home prior to their exam.

There is an important point buried in that last paragraph. Although adults and older children will usually read through an entire line on an eye chart without much prompting or instruction, younger children may need help. You may need to occasionally get off your chair, walk to the eye chart, and point to specific letters with your finger or a pointer.

If a child is young enough that he can't do the "H-O-T-V" chart, the next one to try is the Allen figure chart. The Allen chart looks like a Snellen chart or "H-O-T-V" chart, but instead of being made up of letters, it's made up of black-and-white schematic pictures of things that should be familiar to a small child. Typical pictures include a man on horseback, a birthday cake, a hand, car, telephone, and a duck, but may vary from clinic to clinic. Like the other charts, pictures get smaller to test better visual acuity. Like the "H-O-T-V" chart, shy kids may benefit from having a sheet on their lap to point to rather than having to say what the figure is. Kids can also be sent home with a sheet to practice with for future visits. The biggest disadvantage to using the Allen chart is that it only measures down to about 20/30 or so. If you are really trying to prove 20/20 vision, you will have to go to the "H-O-T-V" or Snellen chart.

If a child isn't old enough to manage the Allen chart or one isn't available, the next one on the list is the "illiterate E" chart, also called the "tumbling E" chart. Although you can use this for children, it is typically used for people who don't speak the same language as the person performing the test. This chart is made up of many versions of the letter "E," which are all pointing in different directions. The "Es" get smaller as we move down the eye chart, just like other systems. All you need to do is ask the patient to point in space (either with one finger or three made to look like an "E") to match the way the fingers of the "E" are pointing.

For very young children (ie, less than a couple of years old), you may need to use Teller acuity cards if you're really trying to record an objective measurement of visual acuity. Teller cards are a stack of cardboard cards that measure about 2 feet long by 1 foot high. One half of each card is blank gray, and the other half has a pattern. Teller cards are based on the idea is that a baby is going to be more interested in looking at a pattern than a blank gray field, and, therefore, should preferentially look at the patterned side. Each card also has a hole in the middle that the tester peeks through from behind to get an accurate idea of which side the patient looks at. Because you are behind the card, it is a "masked" test to give—you don't know which side has the pattern before you present it to your patient. As long as the patient keeps looking at the pattern sides, you keep presenting cards with finer and finer patterns. Eventually, the patient will not be able to differentiate between the pattern side and the gray side, and you can stop. The resulting visual acuity is written on the card.

The Teller acuity cards are a good way to get a visual acuity measurement on a baby or toddler, but a lot of times you don't need to go that far to get a good assessment of visual function. Often it is important merely to know if the child prefers one eye to the other, or if he likes them both equally. In order to see which eye a child prefers, you have to make sure that the two eyes are looking at two different things. If the child comes in with strabismus, you don't need to do anything special. Show the child a target, and then cover one eye. If he has to move the uncovered eye to look at the target, we know he had been looking with the other eye (the one that is now covered). When you take the cover away, if he shifts his eyes back, he clearly prefers the one that was covered. If he does not shift back, he may just be able to alternate meaning that he likes the 2 eyes equally. Then the test is be repeated by covering then uncovering the other eye in the same manner.

A similar test can be done for children without strabismus; you just have to create an artificial strabismus using a prism. If you place a 4^Δ prism base down in front of one of your patient's eyes, you'll create a situation where one eye is looking at one object and the other eye is looking at something else. Then, continue as was described for patients with strabismus. Cover one eye, and see if the eyes move to pick up fixation with the other eye. Then, uncover the first eye, and see if the fixation switches back. In this way, you can determine if he prefers to use one eye over the other. This technique often proves to be the best in managing a young child with amblyopia, also known as a lazy eye. It can be more useful than trying to get an objective measurement of visual acuity using Teller cards or any of the eye charts.

Slit Lamp Examination

Even younger children can be coerced into a slit lamp. With the little ones, this is easiest if they are sitting on their parent's lap. This way, they get all the comfortable, cozy security of sitting on their parent, and also get the elevation that you need to fit them into the slit lamp. Real little, shy, or scared ones may not put their face up to the standard slit lamp. For these children, the portable slit lamp is a useful alternative. This device has the same optics and magnification as a regular slit lamp, but can be held in the examiner's hand. This way, you can bring the slit lamp to the patient rather than bringing the patient to the slit lamp.

Intraocular Pressure

A word about intraocular pressure. I do not typically measure intraocular pressures on children as a matter of routine. They tend to squeeze and be scared, and this produces too many false negatives. However, I do check pressures on every child if there's a specific reason for it, like if there is uveitis, Axenfeld's anomaly, or a history of trauma. Children who can sit at a slit lamp can almost always tolerate Goldmann applanation tonometry. For those who just can't manage it, a tonopen is usually a good alternative. Remember that if a child is crying, even if you can get a measurement with the tonopen, it may likely be artifactually high secondary to the squeezing of the lids.

Examination Under Anesthesia

If a child is very difficult to examine, so much so that you just can't trust the data that you are getting, and there is a problem that needs to be evaluated, do not forget that you can do the exam under anesthesia as a last resort. Remember, you lose your subjective data by doing this. You cannot check for visual acuity or motilities while the child is under anesthesia. However, if you are trying to follow an anatomic problem, such as cataract, a corneal ulcer, or glaucoma, this can sometimes be more easily performed while the child is asleep. Remember that the intraocular pressure will decrease while the patient is under anesthesia, so be sure to check this immediately after the anesthesiologist has put him under.

Basic Optics

In order to begin answering the question "What can or can't my patient see?", you will need to have at least a rudimentary understanding of optics. Optics is the study of the behavior of light. When traveling through the vacuum of space, light travels in a straight line at the speed of light. However, when it travels through something that is denser than the vacuum of space (eg, air, water, plastic, or glass), it will slow down. The denser the material it is traveling through, the more it will slow down. Thus, it will travel slower in plastic than air.

All the interesting things happen when light passes across an interface separating two different materials. Another way to say this is that all the interesting things happen at surfaces—the surface of a lake or a lens. At this surface, some of the light will bounce back (reflection), but more importantly, much of it will be bent (refraction). In the eye clinic, we spend the overwhelming majority of our time interested in how light is bent (refracted) as it crosses the surface separating one material (usually air) and another (usually plastic, glass, or the surface of the eye).

To help simplify the study of optics, we draw light rays as arrows. This is helpful in showing us where the light is coming from, and where it is going to. This system is important in another way, also. By drawing more than one ray of light (arrow) in a beam, we can look at how the different rays are acting in relationship to the other rays within the same beam (Figure 3-1). The rays can spread out, making the beam weaker over time (like the beam of a flashlight) in a situation called *divergence*. The rays can also get closer together over time, making it brighter. This is called *convergence*. If the rays are neither diverging, nor converging, they are *parallel*.

The study of how these light rays are behaving is called *optics*. The behavior of light, whether it's diverging, converging, or parallel, is called *vergence*. Vergence is something that can be measured, and math can be used to study it. Because we can use math, we can use negative and positive signs to help us define things. When light is parallel, there is no vergence, so the vergence

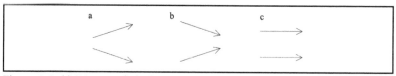

Figure 3-1. (a) Diverging light (minus vergence). (b) Coverging light (plus vergence). (c) Parallel light (vergence=0).

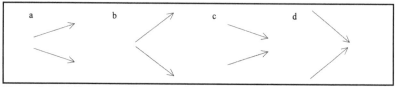

Figure 3-2. (a) Shows a small amount of divergence (maybe –1.00 D), while (b) shows more divergence (maybe –4.00 D). (c) Shows a small amount of convergence (maybe +1.00 D), while (d) shows D convergence (maybe +4.00 D). The closer the rays are to parallel, the smaller the value of the vergence. Parallel light has vergence=0.

equals zero. When light is diverging, it is getting weaker with time, and the vergence is recorded as a negative number. When light is converging, it is getting stronger with time, and the vergence is a positive number.

The unit of measurement for vergence is called the *diopter,* and is abbreviated with a capital letter D. The more the rays of light are diverging or converging, the greater the vergence, and the higher the value in diopters (4 D compared to 1 D, for instance) (Figure 3-2).

Light is created in nature in a diverging fashion. To understand this, think of how you drew the sun when you were in kindergarten. The rays go out from the sun in a diverging manner. The farther you get from the sun (or light bulb, or flashlight) the weaker and more spread out the light becomes. The vergence decreases more and more the farther you travel from the source of the light. Another way to say this is that the greater the distance you are from the point source of light, the less the vergence there will be. The mathematical equation links distance (measured in meters) to vergence (measured in diopters) in an inverse relationship. The formula is simply this:

$$\text{(Vergence in D)} = 1/\text{(Distance in meters)}, \text{ or}$$
$$\text{(Distance in meters)} = 1/\text{(Vergence in D)}$$

It's a reciprocal relationship (one thing = 1/the other) because as one increases (distance) the other decreases (vergence). As we travel farther and farther away from the source of the light, the distance will approach infinity. Mathematically, the vergence, which is 1/distance, will approach zero, because $1/\infty = 0$. A nonmathematical way of describing this is to say that the farther we get from a point source of light, the closer to parallel that

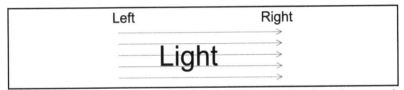

Figure 3-3. It is the convention in light ray diagrams that light is always drawn traveling from left to right.

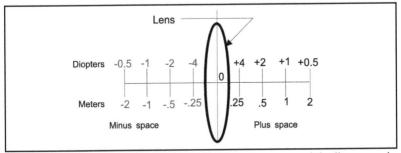

Figure 3-4. All space to the left of the lens is called minus space while all space to the right of the lens is called plus space. The distance from the lens can be measured in vergence in diopters (D) or distance in meters (m) where m=1/D and D=1/m.

light will become. If we move far enough away from the light source, it will become parallel. Mathematically, "far enough away" is defined as "infinity." Practically, "far enough away" is described as 20 feet or 6 meters away, which is why 20 feet is the distance away from the patient where we place the eye chart.

So, to review. Light is created in nature in a diverging manner. The farther we get from the source, the less diverging it will become, until it eventually we will be so far away that the light rays will be parallel. Converging light is not found anywhere in nature. To get converging light, we have to either pass it through a lens, or bounce it off a concave mirror.

Light Ray Diagrams

The next step in understanding optics is to understand the conventions involved in light ray diagrams. For the most part, light ray diagrams will follow certain rules.

1. In light ray diagrams, light rays are represented as arrows that usually travel from left to right (Figure 3-3).

2. The light ray diagram represents a sort-of 2-dimensional graph, where the lens is (almost) always placed at zero (Figure 3-4).

3. Distances from the lens are always measured in meters (m) and vergence is measured in D. A diopter, remember, is merely 1/(distance in meters). (see Figure 3-4).

Figure 3-5. A +2.00 diopter lens (a) will focus parallel light to a point 1/2 m to the right of it, while a +1.00 lens (b) will focus parallel light to a point 1 m to the right of it.

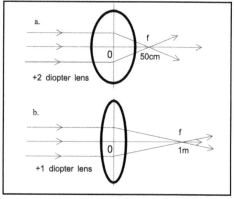

4. All space to the left of the lens is minus space. All distances from the lens are thus recorded as minus numbers and are always written in *red*. Because (as in rule 1) light travels from left to right, it only makes sense that objects are put on the left side—the minus side—of the charts, because light typically is created by the object. This is consistent with everything we've said so far because the object is acting as the point source, and thus must be producing diverging light. If the light is diverging, it has minus vergence, and therefore its source (the object) should be on the minus side of the diagram.

5. All space to the right of the lens is plus space. All distances from the lens are thus recorded as plus numbers and always written in *black* (or blue, white, or some other non-red color).

6. If an image is created on the plus side of the diagram, it is a *real* image. Real images can be visualized by projecting them onto a screen.

7. If an image ends up on the minus side of the diagram, it is a *virtual* image. Virtual images cannot be projected onto a screen, and instead seem to appear within lenses or mirrors.

8. *Parallel* light that enters a lens will be focused at that lens' focal point. The location of the focal point depends upon the lens' power in D. For instance, a +2.00 D lens will focus parallel light 2.00 D away in plus space. Two D works out to be 1/2 meter, or 50 cm. The *higher* that a lens' power is, the *greater* the number of D, and the *closer* to the lens that parallel light will be focused (remember m=1/D) (Figure 3-5).

9. A *plus* lens is any lens that focuses parallel light on the *plus* side of the lens (usually as a real image). Plus lenses are also known as *converging* lenses (because they cause parallel light to converge), or *convex* lenses. The term "plus lens" is the easiest to remember, however, and in keeping with the convention described in #5 above, plus lenses are usually colored black (Figure 3-6).

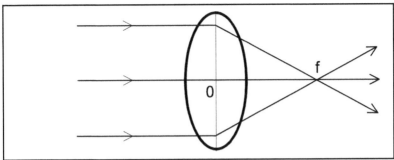

Figure 3-7. A minus lens will usually form an upright, minified, virtual image in minus space.

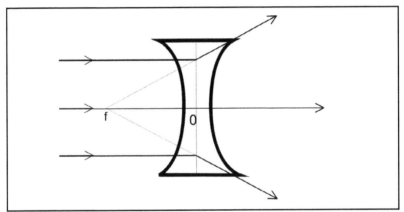

Figure 3-6. A plus lens usually will form an inverted, magnified, real image in plus space.

10. A *minus* lens is any lens that focuses parallel light onto the *minus* side of the lens (usually as a virtual image). Minus lenses are also known as *diverging* lenses (because they cause parallel light to diverge), or *concave* lenses. The term "minus lens" is the easiest to remember, however, and in keeping with the convention described in #4 above, minus lenses are usually colored red (Figure 3-7).

That should be enough basic optics to get you started. To apply optics to the eye clinic, you only need to add a few specific rules.

THE EYE AS AN OPTICAL SYSTEM

In the eye clinic, for light to be considered parallel, it must come from at least 20 feet (or 6 meters) away. This is why our lanes are so long, and thus the birth of the name "lane"—that they look more like country lanes than actual rooms.

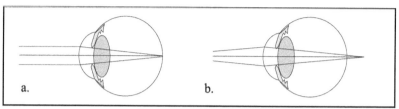

Figure 3-8. An emmetrope will focus parallel light (a) to a point on the retina, but will focus diverging light to a point behind the retina (b).

When considering the eye, the "lens" in our lens diagram is replaced by the entire "refractive apparatus" of the eye. For the most part, this refractive apparatus is the combined optical power of the cornea and crystalline lens. The focal point of this system, hopefully, lies on the retina, because this will allow the patient to see things in focus. Because the retina is typically around 23 mm from the front surface of the cornea, and we know that vergence = (1/distance), it is easy to figure out the total refractive power of the eye as 1/[.023 m] = 43.5 D.

The cornea is the primary refractive contributor of the eye. Refractive surgeons are aware of this and prefer to do surgery on the cornea. Because the cornea is the largest contributor to the refractive power of the eye, a small change in corneal curvature can lead to a large change in the patient's refraction.

Emmetropia

If *parallel* light is focused to a single point on a patient's retina, that patient is labeled emmetropic (Figure 3-8). Emmetropic patients do not need correction to see things that are 20 feet away or greater. If you were to give him an eyeglasses prescription, you would give a spherical lens with power of zero. We don't say "zero," though, when describing this type of lens—all "zero-power" lenses are referred to as *plano*. Thus, emmetropes see objects greater than 20 feet away in sharp focus with plano correction.

However, emmetropes in the relaxed state focus *diverging* light behind the retina (Figure 3-8). You may ask yourself, "When would an emmetrope ever have to focus diverging light?" The simple answer is, "Whenever he looks at anything closer than 20 feet away." Therefore, in a relaxed state, near objects are out of focus for emmetropes. To overcome this diverging light, and thus effectively focus the image onto the retina, the emmetrope must add plus power to the natural refractive power of his eye. If he is young enough, he can accomplish this by *accommodating*. Accommodation adds plus power to the crystalline lens by making it fatter and rounder. In this way, he can change his usual 14 D lens into a 17 D lens and, thus, focus diverging light onto his retina. An older emmetrope has a less flexible crystalline lens and, therefore, needs to wear reading glasses to provide the extra plus power needed to focus near objects on the patient's retina. We will get into this in much greater detail in Chapter 6.

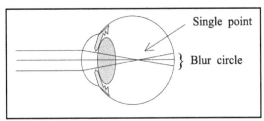

Figure 3-9. A myope focuses light to a single point in the vitreous. What gets projected to the retina is a blur circle. The size of this circle is a major factor in the visual acuity.

A patient who is not emmetropic is called ametropic. The mnemonic is that "emmetrope" begins with the letter "E" because they can see the "E" on the eye chart. Spherical ametropes fall into two classes, *myopes* (near-sighted) and *hyperopes* (far-sighted). Nonspherical ametropes are called *astigmats*. To keep things simple, we'll continue the discussion of ametropia with the spherical examples.

Myopia (Near-Sightedness)

If the refractive power of the eye is too strong, or the eye is too long (or some combination of the two), parallel light is focused in front of the retina—up in the vitreous. What gets projected onto the retina, is a circle instead of a point. This circle is called the *blur-circle*, and the image is perceived by the patient as blurry or fuzzy. This occurs in patients who have *myopia*, also known as near-sightedness (Figure 3-9).

Myopes learn to squint at an early age to see better at distance. In squinting, myopes enlist a natural pinhole effect, much like the pinhole camera or the pinhole device in your examination lane. Because the pinhole is so little, it can circumvent the refractive optics of the eye and allow any myope (or hyperope or astigmat, for that matter) to decrease the size of the blur circle on the retina. Remember Snell's Law: light will only be bent when going from one medium to another if it enters the second medium in any way *other than perpendicularly*. The pinhole takes advantage of this loophole in Snell's Law. It works by only letting light that hits the middle of the cornea reach the cornea at all. All other light is blocked by the material around the pinhole. The light that is allowed to pass through the pinhole is perpendicular (and near perpendicular) to the corneal surface at that point, and therefore does not rely on any refractive properties of the cornea, and is viewed in focus. The light that is blocked by the pinhole device is the light that would have hit the cornea off-center and thus nonperpendicularly (Figure 3-10). This light would have needed to rely upon the cornea and lens to bend it in to focus on the retina, and in a myope, this light would have been focused up in the vitreous instead. Because squinting is really the only tool young myopes can use to see better at distance, they learn to squint at an early age. Usually, this is noticed by parents and teachers, and myopic children are sent to the eye doctor for evaluation while still quite young—usually in grade school.

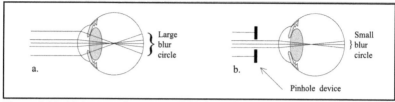

Figure 3-10. (a) A myope focuses parallel light in the vitreous, resulting in a blur circle being projected to the retina. (b) If a pinhole device is placed in front of the cornea, the peripheral incoming light is blocked, and a smaller blur circle is formed resulting in better visual acuity.

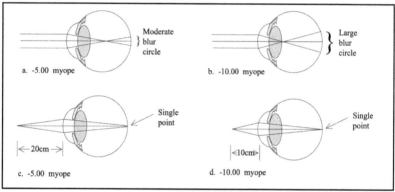

Figure 3-11. (a) A –5.00 D myope will form a smaller blur circle on the retina than a –10.00 D myope (b) when focusing parallel light from an object greater than 20 feet away, and thus, a –5.00 D myope has better distance visual acuity than a –10.00 D myope (although much worse than an emmetrope). (c) A –5.00 D myope sees things in perfect focus when they are positioned 20 cm away, (d) while a –10.00 D myope sees things in perfect focus when they are positioned 10 cm away.

Myopes do well when looking at near objects, and thus the term "nearsightedness" (Figure 3-11). Typically, a myope will best see an object at one specific near distance. When viewing objects at 20 feet away or more, the parallel light is focused in front of the retina, and a blurred image is seen as described above. However, as the object is brought closer to the myope, it comes into sharper and sharper focus. This occurs because the viewed light from the object becomes more and more divergent as the object is brought closer (remember that vergence=1/distance). The more divergent the light becomes, the farther back in the vitreous it is focused. While this occurs, the blur circle on the retina becomes smaller and smaller. Eventually, the object is moved close enough to the eye that the light from the object is focused precisely on the retina, the blur circle becomes a point, the image is perceived as being in focus, and visual acuity is maximized. Where this

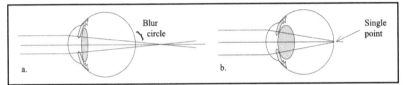

Figure 3-12. (a) A hyperope focuses parallel light to a point behind the retina, resulting in a blur circle being projected onto the retina, and the visual acuity being decreased. (b) By accommodating, a hyperope can fatten his crystalline lens, and may be able to bring parallel light to focus as a single point upon his retina.

occurs depends upon the level of the patient's myopia (remember that distance=1/vergence). Thus, a –5.00 D myope will clearly see an object 20 cm away [distance=1/(5D) = 1/5 m = 20 cm], while a –10.00 D myope will clearly see the same object at 10 cm away [distance = 1/(10D) = 1/10 m = 10 cm]. The more myopic a patient is, the closer he must hold things to see them clearly, and thus the more *near*-sighted he is (see Figure 3-9).

Hyperopia (Far-Sightedness)

If the refractive power of the eye is too weak, or the eye is too short (or a combination of the two), parallel light will be focused behind the retina, in the choroid or sclera. Again, what gets projected onto the retina is a blur circle instead of a single point of light, and the retinal image is blurred. When this occurs, the patient is labeled hyperopic or "far-sighted."

Young hyperopes, unlike young squinting myopes, typically do not need to squint or wear glasses at an early age unless their hyperopia is excessively high, or associated with a strabismus, amblyopia, or excessive astigmatism. Because of this, most young hyperopes aren't caught and put in glasses in grade school like myopes are. Instead, they overcome their hyperopia by making their crystalline lenses fatter, and in this way increase the overall refractive power of their eye. This lens-fattening is called *accommodation*—the same function that allows emmetropes to see things at less than 20 feet away clearly (Figure 3-12). Because people's ability to accommodate decreases with age (hence the need for bifocals and reading glasses as we get older), mild hyperopes often will get their first pair of glasses somewhere in their mid-30s or early 40s. They typically complain more while looking at things up close, because looking at diverging light requires more accommodation than the usual baseline accommodation needed for distance viewing. Because of this, aging hyperopes usually will have an easier time viewing at distance, and hyperopia is known as "*far*-sightedness."

Astigmatism

I will limit this discussion to regular astigmatism, which is usually correctable with a good refraction, and I'll stay away from irregular astigmatism

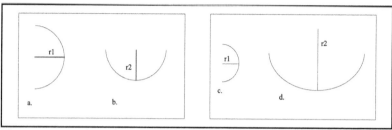

Figure 3-13. A spherical cornea as seen from the side (a) and the top (b). Note that r1=r2, and that the curvature is the same regardless of how the cornea is viewed. An astigmatic cornea as seen from the side (c) and the top (d). Note that r1 does not equal r2, and that the cornea looks different when viewed from the top compared to when it is viewed from the side.

which is not easily correctable, and usually results from pathology (like keratoconus) or prior surgery (like corneal transplant).

The refractive power of a given eye may not be completely symmetrical—that is, it may be more myopic in one area than another, more hyperopic in one area than another, or even myopic in one area and hyperopic in another. It may be that parallel light that hits the cornea near the top (the 12 o'clock position) may be focused one millimeter in front of the retina, while parallel light that hits the cornea near the side (the 9 o'clock position) may be focused 2 mm behind the retina.

If the cornea were perfectly round, like a basketball cut in half, then no matter where parallel light hit, it would all be focused in the same place. If the patient were an emmetrope, it would be focused at a single point on the retina. If the patient were a myope, it would be focused at a single point in front of the retina. If the patient were a hyperope, it would be focused at a single point behind the retina.

Now, let's say the cornea is not perfectly round. Let's say it is shaped not like half a basketball, but more like a football cut in half along its long axis (ie, along the laces). Now you have a cornea that is made up of different curvatures. The least steep curvature is parallel to the long axis of the ball, the direction in which the laces lie. The steepest curvature is perpendicular to the long axis, and lies in the direction your fingers take when you hold it to throw it. In between these two curvatures is an infinite number of intermediate curvatures that slowly increase from the flattest to the steepest.

Let's quickly compare this half-football shaped cornea to a half-basketball shaped one. The half-basketball shaped cornea, representing the spherical system, looks the same whether you stand above your patient looking down, or stand next to him looking from the side (Figure 3-13). No matter from what view you look at your patient's cornea, it always looks the same. This is not so for our regularly astigmatic half-football shaped cornea. If the half-football is lying down, when we look at it from the side, it appears very

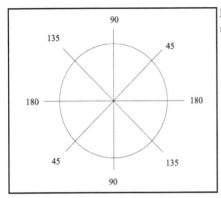

Figure 3-14. The conventional map to record axis of astigmatism.

steep, but when we look at it from the top, it does not appear steep at all. Another patient may have his half-football standing up (awaiting the kickoff, if you will). In this case, it will look steep when viewed from the top, but look shallow when viewed from the side.

What makes things easier for us is the idea that the 2 axes of regular astigmatism are always perpendicular to one other. This will become clearer when we discuss cylindrical and toric systems later in this chapter.

A system has been developed to enable us to map this all out (Figure 3-14). Looking from the front, the eye is round, so we use a variation of the basic 360 degree system. The variation comes in because we only have to go up to 180 degrees because the football always spans the whole cornea, rather than stopping and doing something different in the middle (a regularly astigmatic cornea looks like half a football, not like half an egg). If the long axis of the half-football (the laces, remember) points up, it also points straight down. If it points toward 2 o'clock, it also points to 8 o'clock. Therefore, not only don't we *need* all 360 degrees, but it would be confusing and not helpful to use them all. Straight up (12 o'clock) is labeled 90 degrees, so straight down is also labeled 90 degrees. Straight over to the left (9 o'clock) is labeled 180 degrees; so straight over to the right (3 o'clock) is labeled 180 degrees. Note that 3 o'clock is labeled 180 degrees, and not 0 degrees as you may expect.

There is just one other bit of terminology that you have to know, and, although I'm not generally an advocate for this type of learning, the best way to learn it is to just memorize it. I am talking about the terminology "with-the-rule" and "against-the-rule." If someone has astigmatism so that his eye is steepest at (or around) 90 degrees (like a football lying down), he is said to have with-the-rule astigmatism. Conversely, if someone has astigmatism so that his cornea is steepest at (or around) 180 degrees (like a football standing up), he is said to have against-the-rule astigmatism. As a general rule,

Figure 3-15. A power cross for the prescription, +1.00 +2.00 × 90, which can also be written as +3.00 –2.00 × 180.

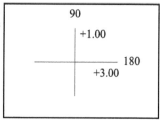

younger people have with-the-rule, and older people have against-the-rule astigmatism—but that's just a general rule. Now that we have our axes, let's put them to good use.

CROSSES AND LENSES

Power Cross

A power cross is used to map out where a patient's axes of astigmatism lie, and what the *power* is along each of these axes. Let's say, for example, that parallel light that goes through a cornea at the 12 o'clock position (90 degrees) is focused behind the retina in such a way that it needs a +1.00 D lens to bring it onto the retina and therefore into focus. Let's also say that in this same eye, parallel light that goes through the cornea at the 9 o'clock position (180 degrees) is focused behind the retina in such a way that it needs a +3.00 D lens to bring it onto the retina as a single point. One way to picture what is going on is with what is called a power cross. To draw a power cross for this patient, place a +1.00 D near the 90 degree mark (up or down doesn't matter), and a +3.00 D near the 180 degree mark (left or right doesn't matter) (Figure 3-15).

It is important to understand that you are not really putting the patient's error on this diagram. What goes there is what lenses it takes to *correct* the patient's error. This makes sense because we are more interested in how we're going to help him, rather than exactly what his underlying problem is.

The astigmatism that the above person has is regular astigmatism, as was stated previously. This tells us a lot of valuable information. First, the +1.00 D is the lowest number that we will find anywhere on this eye. Second, the +3.00 D is the highest number that we will find. Third, the +1.00 D and +3.00 D are always 90 degrees apart (we treat half-footballs, not half-eggs). Fourth, if you take a point half way between the two axes, at 45 degrees (or 135 degrees), the power there would be +2.00 D (which is halfway between +1.00 and +3.00 D).

This brings us to the idea of the *spherical equivalent*. We'll go into this in more detail again, but at this stage, the spherical equivalent should be thought of as this person's average correction. If you look at the correction needed to bring parallel light into focus at an infinite number of places on this

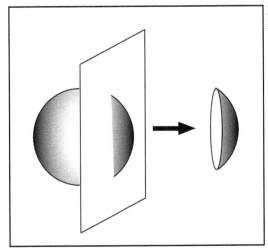

Figure 3-16. A spherical lens is cut from a glass sphere.

eye, and average them together, you'd end up with the spherical equivalent. There are two ways to come up with someone's spherical equivalent. One way is to average the lowest and highest numbers on the lens diagram [in this example, that would be ½ (1.00 + 3.00) = 2.00]. A second way is to add half the difference between the highest and lowest numbers to the lowest number [1.00 + ½ (3.00 − 1.00) = 2.00]. Which way you decide to calculate it will depend on what how the data is presented to you. Regardless of how you calculate it though, the result should always come out the same.

Spherical Lenses

Spherical plus lenses are just that, lenses cut from glass spheres (Figure 3-16). Think of them as having a curved front surface (from the sphere), and a flat back surface (from where it was cut). Light passing through a spherical lens will be focused to a point. Where that point lies depends on that lens' power (distance=1/vergence) and the divergent or convergent nature of the incoming light. A more powerful lens will focus light closer to itself than a less powerful one. Likewise, a plus lens will focus converging light closer to itself than it will parallel light. And that same lens, naturally, will focus diverging light farther away than either parallel or converging light. At this point, you don't need to know any more about spherical lenses other than what was discussed above in the section on light ray diagrams. Basically, spherical lenses are what you think of when you think of lenses.

Cylindrical Lenses

Cylindrical lenses are lenses cut from glass cylinders (Figure 3-17). They are always cut parallel to the long axis of the cylinder. When light passes

Figure 3-17. A cylindrical lens is cut from a glass cylinder.

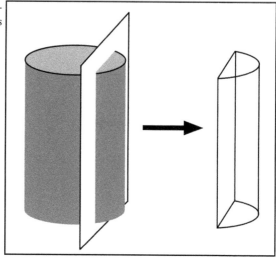

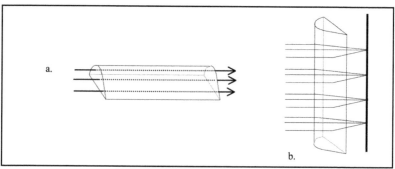

a.

b.

Figure 3-18. (a) When parallel light passes through a cylindrical lens parallel to that lens' long axis, it is not bent at all; it exits the lens as parallel light. (b) When parallel light passes through a cylindrical lens perpendicular to its long axis, it is focused to a line.

through a cylindrical lens parallel to its long axis, it is not bent at all (Figure 3-18). It both enters and exits the lens perpendicularly to a cut surface, and therefore (remember Snell's Law), the light isn't bent at all. When light passes through a cylindrical lens perpendicularly to its long axis, it is focused to a line.

To prove that light is focused to a line, pick up a plus cylindrical lens from your lens tray and shine a light through it. If you don't have a lens tray, consult Figure 3-19. A cylindrical lens can be thought of as a group of two-dimensional wedge-shaped lenses stacked on top of one another. Each infinitely thin wedge-shaped lens focuses parallel light to a point. Because these wedges are stacked one atop the other, all of these points stack up to form a line.

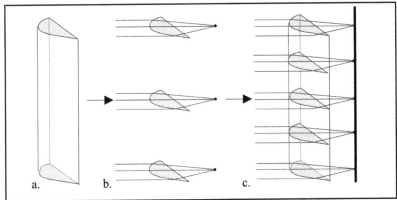

Figure 3-19. A cylindrical lens (a) can be thought of as a stack of infinitely thin crescent-shaped lenses (b) that all focus parallel light to a point. When these crescent-shaped lenses are stacked into a cylinder, their stacked focal points form a focal line (c).

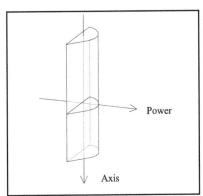

Figure 3-20. The long-axis of a cylindrical lens is called the axis of that lens. Parallel light is focused to a line parallel to the axis. The power of the lens is perpendicular to the long axis of the lens.

At this point, it is important to reiterate this important difference between spherical and cylindrical lenses: *Spherical lenses focus light to a point while cylindrical lenses focus light to a line.* The direction of the line that a cylindrical lens focuses light to is the *axis* of that lens (Figure 3-20). The axis is not dependent upon the actual lens itself, but just on how you happen to hold it. Spherical lenses, of course, have no axis because they cannot focus light to a line, and therefore it doesn't matter how you hold them.

What happens if light is passed through a cylindrical lens in the direction of its axis? Nothing. Remember Figure 3-18. Light passing through a cylindrical lens parallel to its long axis is not bent in any way; it is just as if there were no lens there at all. Therefore, in the direction of a cylinder lens' axis, there is absolutely no *power*. All of the power of a cylindrical lens is perpendicular to its axis. Light is bent most when it passes through a cylindrical lens exactly perpendicular to its axis. This is a very important

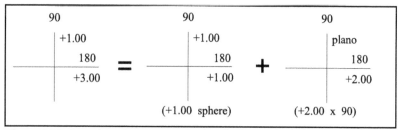

Figure 3-21. An astigmatic system can be described as a spherical and plus cylindrical lens. Here, a +1.00 spherical lens is added to a +2.00 cylindrical lens held axis 90. The resulting astigmatic (toric) lens is written as the combination: +1.00 +2.00 × 90.

but peculiar relationship specific to cylindrical lenses. When we describe a cylindrical lens, we refer to it in terms of its axis and power. These are all the data needed for any given cylindrical lens, yet in the direction of the axis, there is no power. The greatest power, the highest light-bending ability of that lens, occurs exactly 90 degrees from its defining axis.

Back to Power Crosses

Let's have another look at our power cross from before (Figure 3-15). As we recall, our patient is corrected with +1.00 D at 90 degrees and +3.00 D at 180 degrees. Because we know that this patient has *regular* astigmatism, we also know that +1.00 D is the lowest correction anywhere (Figure 3-21). Therefore, we can put up a +1.00 D spherical lens and be certain that we won't be overcorrecting anywhere. With a +1.00 D spherical lens up there, what do we have left that we need to correct? At 90 degrees, we have corrected everything. At 180 degrees, we still need to correct +2.00 D (+3.00 D minus the +1.00 D of the spherical lens). We obviously can't put up an additional +2.00 spherical lens to correct the error at 180 degrees, because that would also give us 2.00 D of power at 90 degrees where we do not need it. But we can correct the remaining error with a cylindrical lens. A +2.00 D cylindrical lens will correct for +2.00 D in the direction of its power, and will correct for zero diopters in the direction of its axis. In this example, we want the zero correction at 90 degrees, so that is the direction of the axis. We want the +2.00 correction at 180 degrees, so that is the direction of the power. Remember that the power and the axis are always 90 degrees apart. Our final correction is "+1.00 D spherical lens with a +2.00 D cylindrical lens held so that its axis lies at 90 degrees." This is wordy, of course, so we have shortened this to the following shorthand: "+1.00 +2.00 × 90." Congratulations, you've just written your first prescription for eyeglasses!

Let's take a minute to look at what we just wrote down as a prescription and make sure we understand what each of the numbers mean. The first number (+1.00) stands alone. This is the spherical lens that is at the base

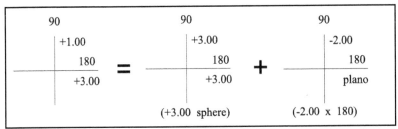

Figure 3-22. An astigmatic system can also be described as a spherical and minus cylindrical lens. Here, a +3.00 spherical lens is added to a −2.00 cylindrical lens held axis 180. The resulting astigmatic (toric) lens is written as the combination: +3.00 −2.00 × 180.

of the correction. The second two numbers go together. The middle one (+2.00) is the *power*, and the last one (90) is the *axis* of the cylindrical lens. Both of these numbers have to work together to describe this cylindrical lens—neither number means anything when it stands alone. So, when we write, "+1.00 +2.00 × 90," we have to remember that we are actually writing "(+1.00) (+2.00 × 90)", just without the parentheses.

Let's do the same exercise, but in a different way (Figure 3-22). Remember our patient was corrected with +1.00 D at 90 degrees, and +3.00 D at 180 degrees. Instead of correcting with a +1.00 sphere like last time, let's put up a +3.00 sphere. We know that the highest correction needed anywhere on that cornea is +3.00, so if we put up a +3.00 sphere, we can't be undercorrecting anywhere. This takes care of the problem at 180 degrees, but brings the image of light passing through the cornea at the 90-degree area to focus up in the vitreous. As a matter of fact, it leaves us needing −2.00 D at 90 degrees to put the image of light passing through there back on to the retina. They make minus cylinder lenses just like they do plus ones. We know we need the full power of that −2.00 cylinder at 90 degrees, and we don't need any power at all at 180 degrees. We align the axis of the cylindrical lens where we need no power, and in this example, that is along the 180-degree meridian. The resultant prescription is "+3.00 D spherical lens with a −2.00 D cylindrical lens held so that its axis lies along the 180 degree meridian." The eyeglasses prescription is written as "+3.00 −2.00 × 180," which really means (+3.00)(−2.00 × 180).

The first way that we solved this patient's refractive problem (+1.00 +2.00 × 90) gave us the prescription in "plus cylinder" notation. It is called "plus cylinder" because it uses a spherical lens, and a plus cylindrical lens. The second way (+3.00 −2.00 × 180) that we solved his problem was written in "minus cylinder" notation. This gets its name because we used a spherical lens and a minus cylindrical lens. In effect, there are 2 ways of saying the same thing. There is an easy 3-step process to convert from plus cylinder notation to minus cylinder notation and back again. Let's

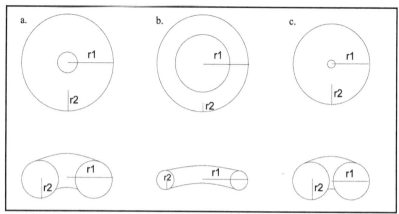

Figure 3-23. Two representations of 3 different toric shapes are shown. The bottom row shows the cross section of each torus positioned directly above it. Each torus is defined by its 2 different radii of curvature. r1 represents the diameter of the doughnut, while r2 represents the height of the doughnut. The r1 of torus(a) equals the r1 of torus (b), but the r2 of these 2 shapes are different. The r2 of torus (a) is equal to the r2 of torus (c), but the r1s are different.

look at our two prescriptions and transpose from plus cylinder (a) to minus cylinder (b):

    a.   +1.00 +2.00 × 90

    b.   +3.00 −2.00 × 180

1. Add the first two numbers of (a) together to get the new sphere – the first number of (b). (+1.00 +2.00 = **+3.00**)
2. Change the sign of the second number of (a) to get the new cylindrical power – the second number of (b). (+2.00 becomes **−2.00**)
3. Add or subtract 90 from the third number in (a) to get the new cylindrical axis – the third number in (b). (90 + 90 = **180**)
4. Put it all together and you get +3.00 −2.00 × 180

The same thing works to go from minus cylinder (b) to plus cylinder (a)

1. +3.00 −2.00 = **+1.00**
2. -2.00 becomes **+2.00**
3. 180 − 90 = **90**
4. Put them together and you get +1.00 +2.00 × 90—which, remember, is really (+1.00) (+2.00 × 90).

Now, up to this point, we have talked about spherical lenses and cylindrical lenses. Spherical lenses are cut from glass spheres, and have the same power everywhere. Cylindrical lenses are cut from glass cylinders, and have an axis with no power, and maximum power 90 degrees away. However, the system described above is neither spherical (the power isn't the same everywhere), nor cylindrical (the power is not plano anywhere). This system is called *toric*, and has more than one power (so it's not spherical), and isn't plano anywhere (so it's not cylindrical).

Just as a spherical lens is cut from a glass sphere, and a cylindrical lens is cut from a glass cylinder, a toric lens is cut from a glass *torus*. A torus is shaped like a doughnut. It has two radii of curvature—the diameter of the doughnut, and the height of the doughnut (Figure 3-23). These two radii of curvature essentially correspond to the powers along the two astigmatic axes of the torus. Another way to think of it is one radius is related to the power of the spherical lens, while the other is related to the power of the cylindrical lens. Patients with astigmatism have toric refractive problems. However, it would be too difficult and cumbersome to try to fix them with toric lenses (we would need an infinite number of toric lenses). Instead, we fix their problems by teasing out the spherical and cylindrical components, and fixing these separately with spherical and cylindrical lenses as we did in the examples above. This is performed through the technique known as *refraction*, which is the subject of the next few chapters.

SAMPLE PROBLEMS WITH ANSWERS

Problems

1. Give prescriptions in minus and plus cylinder based on the following astigmatic cross diagram.

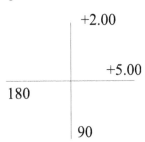

2. Give a plus cylinder correction for the following patient:

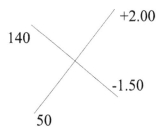

3. Give a minus cylinder correction for the following patient:

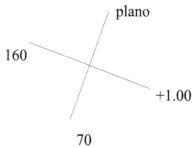

4. Transpose −3.00 +6.00 × 45 to minus cylinder.
5. Transpose −3.00 −6.00 × 105 to plus cylinder.
6. Transpose plano +1.50 × 90 to minus cylinder.
7. Transpose −4.50 sphere to minus cylinder.
8. What is the spherical equivalent of −2.00 +1.50 × 180?
9. What is the spherical equivalent of −2.00 −1.50 × 180?
10. What is the spherical equivalent of this patient:

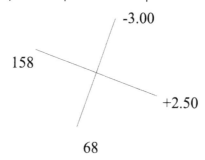

11. Draw a power cross diagram for the patient with correction −3.00 +1.00 × 90.

12. Draw a power cross diagram for the patient with correction +3.00 −3.00 × 45.

Answers

1. Plus cylinder:
   a. The lowest correction needed is +2.00, so let's start with a +2.00 sphere.
   b. We'll need a cylindrical lens to fix the remaining areas. We need +3.00 more diopters with its power at 180 (or, a +3.00 D cylinder with its axis at 90).
   c. Put them together, and you get +2.00 +3.00 x90.

Minus cylinder way:

    a. The highest correction needed is +5.00, so let's start with a *+5.00* sphere.

    b. We'll need a cylindrical lens to fix the remaining areas. We need to take away 3.00 D of power at 90 (or add a −3.00 D cylinder with its axis at *180*).

    c. Put them together, and you get +5.00 −3.00 × 180.

2. Don't let the fact that our axes are not at 90 and 180 degrees worry you. The important thing is that they're 90 degrees apart (140 − 50 = 90).

    a. The lowest correction is −1.50, so we'll put up a *−1.50* sphere.

    b. That leaves 3.50 D of power needed at 50 degrees [+2.00 −(−1.50)= +3.50], so we need to add a *+3.50* cylinder with its axis at *140*.

    c. Put them all together to get −1.50 +3.50 × 140.

3. Again, don't let the weird axes bother you. Also, remember that plano is another way of saying zero.

    a. The highest correction is +1.00, so put up a *+1.00* sphere.

    b. Now you'll need to put up −1.00 D of cylinder with its power at 70 degrees, or *−1.00* D with axis of *160* degrees.

    c. Put them together to get +1.00 −1.00 x160.

4. We start with −3.00 +6.00 × 45.

    a. Add -3.00 to +6.00 to get *+3.00*.

    b. Reverse the sign of +6.00 to get *−6.00*.

    c. Add 90 to 45 to get *135*.

    d. Put it all together to get: +3.00 −6.00 × 135.

5. We start with −3.00 −6.00 x105.

    a. Add −3.00 to −6.00 to get *−9.00*.

    b. Reverse the sign of −6.00 to get *+6.00*.

    c. Subtract 90 from 105 to get *15*.

    d. Put it all together to get: −9.00 +6.00 × 15.

6. We start with plano +1.50 × 90.

    a. Add plano (zero) to +1.50 to get *+1.50*.

    b. Reverse the sign of +1.50 to get *−1.50*.

    c. Add 90 to 90 to get *180*.

    d. Put it all together to get: +1.50 −1.50 × 180.

7. This is a trick question. It's a spherical correction, so there is no cylinder. Therefore you can't really write it in plus or minus cylinder.

8. Because you know the prescription formula, it's easiest to find the spherical equivalent this way: −2.00 + ½(1.50) = −1.25.

9. Ditto. -2.00 + ½(−1.50) = −2.75.

10. Because you know the power at the two main axes, and don't know the actual eyeglasses prescription (although I'm sure you could easily figure it out), it's easiest to find the spherical equivalent this way: ½(−3.00 + 2.50) = −0.25. Because this patient has *regular* astigmatism, −0.25 is also the power exactly halfway between the two main axes (at axis 113 and 23).

11.

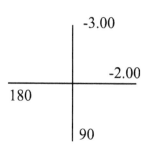

12.

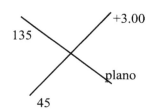

4

Subjective Refraction

Refraction is the cornerstone of what we do. As eye care professionals, one of our fundamental duties is to help patients to see better, and the vast majority of the time, this can be managed simply with an accurate refraction. Refraction can be performed with loose, hand-held lenses and trial frames, but if you're new to the eye clinic, the phoropter is probably the best way to start out.

VISUAL ACUITY

In understanding refraction it is helpful to understand what is meant by the term "visual acuity." Best visual acuity is obtained when light that enters the eye is focused directly onto the retina at a single point. As you recall from Chapter 3, this situation occurs whenever an emmetrope looks at something that is greater than 20 feet away. However, remember that for the uncorrected myope or hyperope, parallel light is focused onto the retina as a circle, and for the uncorrected astigmat, it is focused there as either a line or (as we will soon see) as a circle or ellipse. Thus, each uncorrected myope, hyperope, and astigmat has decreased distance visual acuity when compared to an uncorrected emmetrope. Fortunately, almost every myope, hyperope, and astigmat can usually be corrected so that light is focused onto his retina at a single point, and thus have the same visual acuity as an emmetrope. This feat can be performed with a technique called *refraction*.

The best way to think of visual acuity is to think of it as similar to a test that neurologists do: 2-point discrimination. This is a test that evaluates receptive fields of nerves. You ask a patient to close his eyes, then touch his skin with 2 mildly sharp objects and ask if he can recognize them as 1 object or 2 (Figure 4-1). In order for the objects to be recognized as 2, they must trigger two separate sensory neurons that, in turn, trigger 2 separate brain nerves. Receptive fields are quite large on the sole of the foot or on the back, so the 2 mildly sharp objects must be far apart before they excite 2 separate brain

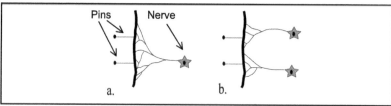

Figure 4-1. (a) In areas like the lower back, neurons have very large receptive fields. If 2 pins are touched to the skin within the receptive field of a neuron, they are perceived as 1 pin. (b) Areas like the fingertips contain neurons with small receptive fields. Here, the 2 pins, although the same distance apart as in (a), are within receptive fields from 2 separate neurons, and are, therefore, perceived as 2.

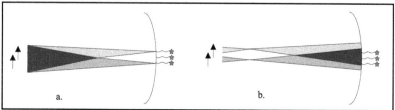

Figure 4-2. (a) For an emmetrope, parallel light from 2 objects is focused to the retina as 2 single points. If these 2 points each stimulate a photoreceptor leaving 1 unstimulated photoreceptor between them, the 2 objects are seen as separate. (b) In the myope displayed here, light from both objects stimulates a number of photoreceptors, and, therefore, they are not perceived as separate.

nerves and, thus, be perceived as 2 separate objects. Receptive fields are quite small on the tip of the tongue and finger and, as a result, the patient can recognize 2 objects as separate when poked here even when the 2 objects are millimeters apart. The retina works similarly.

Visual acuity is a function of central vision that falls under the jurisdiction of the macula. Let's forget, for a minute, all the cross-linking of neurons in the middle layers of the retina, and say that each photoreceptor in the macula has a direct line to an individual neuron in the visual cortex of the brain. If this were true, the brain would be able to differentiate between when one photoreceptor fires and the one right next to it does not. Remember that in the case of the emmetrope, parallel light is focused onto the retina at a single point. Theoretically, that point should be small enough to hit only one photoreceptor while missing the ones on either side (Figure 4-2). That being the case, an emmetrope should be able to differentiate 2 objects when they are held quite close together. In fact, an emmetrope should be able to recognize 2 objects with only 3 photoreceptors being involved. This occurs if the light from the first object is focused to excite the first photoreceptor; the light from the second object is focused to excite the third photoreceptor; and the second photoreceptor is not excited. Don't underestimate the importance

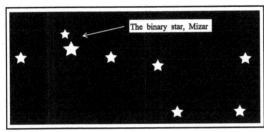

The binary star, Mizar

Figure 4-3. Hundreds of years ago, Native Americans used the binary star, Mizar, as a nonquantitative measurement of visual acuity.

of this second, unexcited, photoreceptor. This photoreceptor is the one that allows an emmetrope to recognize the 2 objects as 2 separate objects by recognizing the space between them. If light from the 2 objects excites 2 adjacent photoreceptors, the objects can not be recognized as separate because the space between them can not be appreciated. The brain will just assume it's seeing a single, bigger object.

The uncorrected ametrope does not focus parallel light onto his retina at a single point. Remember the myope who focuses light to a point up in his vitreous, and thus light is projected onto his retina as a circle called a blur circle. Remember also the hyperope who focuses light to a single point back in his choroid or sclera, and thus light is also projected onto his retina as a blur circle. Remember also the astigmat, who focuses light in strange ways still to be discussed, but take it as said that light is projected onto his retina as either a line, ellipse or circle. In all of these cases, many more than one photoreceptor will be triggered whenever parallel light is focused onto the retina. Each object may excite 2, 5, 10, or even 100s or 1000s photoreceptors. To be perceived as separate, 2 objects here must be moved far enough apart that the blur circles be completely separated by a row of photoreceptors that are not triggered. The larger the blur circles, the farther apart their centers must be, and therefore the farther apart the viewed objects must be if they are to be perceived as separate.

Visual acuity is really little more than measuring how close together these two objects can be held while still being perceived as separate. You can actually measure visual acuity by directly measuring 2-point discrimination. It is an easy enough thing to do. Some Native American tribes supposedly used the stars to perform a similar test of visual acuity (Figure 4-3). Young tribes people were tested to establish whether or not they could recognize both stars of the binary star, Mizar, in the handle of the Big Dipper. This test was a fairly selective one, as the two stars are separated by about ten seconds of arc when viewed from the surface of the earth. Its basic limitation, of course, is that it wasn't a quantitative test—either a tribesperson could see the 2 stars or he could not.

You don't need 2 stars held that many light years away to measure visual acuity utilizing a system of 2-point discrimination. In fact, all you need are 2-small objects and a 20-foot long room. While standing 20 feet from your patient, hold 2 small objects together. Then, slowly, move the 2 objects away

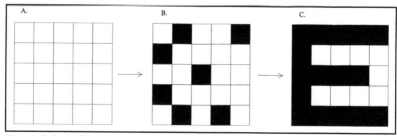

Figure 4-4. Snellen letters are merely a specific form of 2-point discrimination. The patient, in a way, is asked to report what squares of 5-x-5 grid are colored black, and which are colored white. This could be done in a random fashion, as in (b), but it is much easier for the patient to report answers when the colored-in squares map out to familiar figures, as in (c).

from one another until the patient says he recognizes them as 2 separate objects. The distance the 2 objects are from each other when they are recognized as separate is a crude measure of that patient's visual acuity.

This method is, of course, unwieldy and difficult to administer in a reproducible way. However, what we actually do in the clinic is based upon just this principle. Think of it this way. Instead of having 2 random objects, place a 5-by-5 square grid 20 feet from your patient (Figure 4-4). You can then fill in various squares in the grid so that the patient must recognize when some of the squares are white, and some are black. Emmetropes should easily see which squares are filled in and which are not. Ametropes can only do so if the squares, and thus the entire grid, are large enough that none of the blur circles overlap (either that, or held closer than 20 feet away). If the squares are colored in correctly, you can make them into familiar symbols like letters (Snellen letters or HOTV) or shapes (Allen figures or "tumbling Es"). Thus, instead of asking your patient which squares are colored in and which are not, you can simply ask which letter or shape is he looking at. For patients who cannot make out which squares are colored and which are not, (who cannot tell you which letter is represented by the grid), you need to get a grid with bigger squares positioned farther apart. This is simply obtained by either using the next bigger grid that conveniently is represented by the next bigger Snellen letter or Allen figure, or moving the current grid closer.

Often, a patient will ask you, "You said I'm 20/50 without glasses and 20/20 with glasses; what does that mean?" I've found that the best way to answer this question is to say, "What you can see at 20 feet away with your glasses off, you can see from 50 feet away with your glasses on."

It must be borne in mind that visual acuity is merely that, visual acuity. It is a very specific and incomplete way of defining how well a patient sees. All visual acuity tells you is how well a patient can discern stationary, black letters from a well-lit, white background positioned 20 feet away. Do not fall

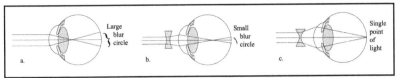

Figure 4-5. (a) An uncorrected myope focuses light far up in the vitreous, resulting in a blur circle of light being projected onto the retina. (b) If a weak minus lens is placed in front of the cornea, diverging light is presented to the cornea, the focal point of the system is moved back in the vitreous, and a smaller blur circle is formed on the retina. (c) When the proper minus lens is found, diverging light hits the cornea so that the light is focused to a single point on the retina, and visual acuity is maximized.

into the trap of assuming they see well just because they have good visual acuity. Many patients with 20/20 or 20/15 visual acuity will tell you that they are frustrated because they feel they cannot see. Complaints of poor vision from any patient with good visual acuity need to be taken seriously, and further evaluation may include contrast sensitivity, visual field testing, color vision, stereopsis, or other specific tests.

REFRACTING THE SPHERICAL MYOPE

The basic idea behind refracting the myope is an easy one. To get the myope to have the same visual acuity as the emmetrope, you have to somehow get him to focus parallel light to a single point on the retina, just like the emmetrope. As discussed previously, the uncorrected myope focuses parallel light to a point up in his vitreous. This occurs because either the refracting apparatus (cornea and lens) is too strong, or the eye is just too long, or, more likely, some combination of the 2. Because the light is focused to a single point in the vitreous, a blur circle rather than a point of light falls on the myope's retina. We demonstrated above how this blur circle results in decreased visual acuity for the myope when compared to the emmetrope or lesser myope and, therefore, the need to be presented with a larger "E" on the eye chart. To correct the myope, we merely need to push the focal point of his refracting system back to his retina. The correction is accomplished with the aid of minus lenses.

Remember that minus lenses cause parallel light to diverge. Diverging light must be bent more than parallel light if it is to focused to a point. Another way to think of this is that the optical system of the eye has a more difficult time bending diverging light than it does parallel light. This extra effort absorbs some of the surplus refracting power of the myope, and allows light to be focused farther back in the vitreous. As stronger and stronger minus lenses are placed in front of the myope's eye, his visual apparatus must bend light of greater and greater divergence, resulting in the light being focused farther and farther back in the vitreous, and the blur circle on the retina becoming smaller and smaller. Eventually, the proper lens is chosen and the

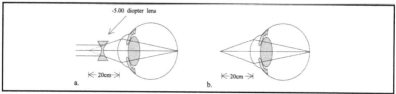

Figure 4-6. This corrected –5.00 D myope (a) is "tricked," with the help of a –5.00 D lens, into thinking that everything held at greater than 20 feet away is really at his ideal near distance. The light hits his cornea with the same amount of divergence as an object held 20 cm away (b).

light is focused to a single point focused squarely on the retina (Figure 4-5), and maximal visual acuity is obtained.

It can really be this simple: You ask a –3.00 myope to read the eye chart. He can only read the 20/150 line. You put up a –1.00 lens, and he can now read the 20/80 line. You put up a –2.00 lens, and he can read the 20/40 line. You put up a –3.00 lens, and he can see the 20/20 line, and you're done.

The idea that a myope sees best when looking at diverging light is not a new one. While this principle is discussed in Chapter 3, it is reviewed here again. Parallel light only comes from objects at least 20 feet from the viewer. Light from any closer object will be diverging when it reaches the patient's eye. Each myope has a specific place up close where viewed objects will appear in focus. For the –1.00 D myope, this point is one meter away, while for the –5.00 D myope, this point falls 20 cm away (m=1/d). When we correct a myope with minus lenses, what we are really doing is tricking him into thinking that everything he looks at off in the distance is in fact at that one close distance away that he likes to hold things (Figure 4-6). The –1.00 D myope is tricked into thinking that everything on the horizon that he looks at is really only one meter away, while the –5.00 D myope is tricked into thinking that everything on the horizon that he looks at is really only 20 cm away. The reason the myope can be tricked in this way is because the glasses we prescribe make parallel light diverge in such a way that it hits the cornea exactly the way light from a close object does when that patient is not wearing his glasses. His cornea cannot tell the difference.

Beware of one thing when refracting people with minus lenses. Minus lenses minify the image, as stated before, and, therefore, they typically make the image appear smaller and darker. For many patients, this "smaller and darker" is incorrectly perceived as sharper even when the visual acuity may have decreased. It is easy to give a patient more minus than needed because you may be continually told that he likes the images seen through the more minus lenses better. The younger patient is especially at risk because when he is over-minused, the image can still be brought into sharp focus. The patient does this by accommodating and allowing himself to recognize even the smallest Snellen letters or Allen figures even though he is looking through the

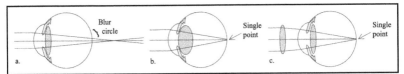

Figure 4-7. An uncorrected, relaxed hyperope (a) will focus parallel light to a single point behind the retina resulting in a blur circle being projected onto the retina. There are 2 ways a hyperope can be corrected. In the first way, (b) the hyperope can help himself by fattening his crystalline lens through accommodation. In the second way, (c) a plus lens can be placed in front of his cornea via spectacles or contact lenses.

incorrect lens. Be aware of this problem. If you think you have over-minused a patient, merely blur him by giving him an extra 1 to 2 D of plus and restart the refraction from that new power. Also, be in the habit of refracting the patient from the plus side, always carefully dialing in more minus, thus moving the image back through his vitreous toward his retina. Try not to refract from the minus side, dialing in plus to move the image forward toward the retina from the scleral side. You will be much more likely to over minus your patient if you proceed in this fashion. By using the proper technique, you will always work against your patient's tendency to accommodate, and thus you will minimize your risk of over-minusing him.

REFRACTING THE SPHERICAL HYPEROPE

As discussed in Chapter 3, the hyperope focuses parallel light to a single point behind the retina because the optical power of the eye is too weak in relation to the length of his eye. The hyperope needs help converging light because his eye just cannot do it alone. We can help him converge by giving a converging lens, otherwise known as a plus lens. As we place stronger and stronger plus lenses in front of the hyperope, the light is focused farther and farther forward toward the retina until eventually it is focused at a single point exactly on the retina. The one plus lens that helps the hyperope focus parallel light directly on his retina is the lens that will provide him with the best visual acuity.

Accommodation is covered in detail in Chapter 6, but at this point, I will describe a little about how accommodation can hurt your ability to accurately refract your patient. Most young people, but especially hyperopes, walk around with a certain amount of what we call, "accommodative tone." What this means is that many of us accommodate at least a little bit all of the time. Remember that accommodation results in a fattening of the crystalline lens of the eye. This fattening increases the plus power of the crystalline lens and, thus, increases the plus power of the optical system of the eye. In the case of the hyperope, this allows for a natural decrease in his refractive error and a natural improvement of his visual acuity (Figure 4-7). This improvement occurs because the uncorrected or undercorrected hyperope focuses light behind the retina, and any force that brings the focal point forward automatically brings it closer to the retina, thus resulting in a smaller blur circle landing on the retina and things appearing in better focus.

The problem, however, occurs when we want to help the hyperope by prescribing glasses. If he is accommodating when we refract him, we will underestimate the total amount of hyperopia that needs to be corrected. For example, look at the +5.00 D hyperope who thinks he is helping you by accommodating 2.00 D during your refraction. In this situation, the patient corrects with only +3.00 D of extra help: +5.00 D (his total error) minus +2.00 (from his accommodation)=+3.00 D (your refraction). In order to like the glasses you give him, he will need to always be accommodating those 2.00 D. This may get tiresome after a while, especially when he reads and needs to enlist an extra 3.00 D of accommodation to bring the reading material into focus (this is elaborated in Chapter 6).

So what can you do to ensure that the patient is not accommodating during the refraction? The first thing you need to remember to do is to refract from the plus side while adding minus lenses. This technique was discussed in the section above on "refracting the myope." It's an important concept, and is useful for preventing your patient from adding more accommodation during his examination. Unfortunately, it's not always enough to overcome his baseline, walking-around accommodative tone.

If you think that you cannot get your patient to stop accommodating during your refraction, you should consider performing the refraction while after he has had cycloplegic, dilating eyedrops. This type of refraction is called a cycloplegic refraction (CR). This is in contrast to a manifest refraction (MR), which is performing a refraction without dilating drops.

If you have a young patient, you should always compare his manifest (without drops) refraction to the cycloplegic refraction. If the two are similar, just give the patient the MR. If the two are different, the CR will usually be more on the plus side than the MR. Unfortunately, you usually can't get away with just giving the patient a CR, the way you can an MR, because you never know exactly how much accommodative tone he needs to be comfortable. As I said before, many people like to walk around with at least a little bit of accommodation all the time. What you need to do is bring him back 1 or 2 weeks later being sure all the cycloplegic has worn off. Then repeat your MR, but "push plus." To push plus, you merely give your patient more plus than he thinks he wants, and give him a couple of minutes to relax accommodation and get used to it. A proper "push-plus" refraction may take a half-hour or more, where the majority of the time the patient is sitting in the waiting room trying to get used to the added power. Continue to give him a little more plus every 5 to 10 minutes until he cannot relax anymore to accept any more plus. Remember that you are not doing this blindly because you know what his CR is and, therefore, know about how much plus you can potentially push before you have reached the limits of your patient's accommodative relaxation. When you think you are done, let the patient walk around with the trial frames on to be sure he likes that prescription before you write it out.

REFRACTING THE ASTIGMAT

Unfortunately, the basic concept behind refracting the astigmat is not an easy one. Actually, that's not exactly true. It's just that conceptualizing the astigmat, in general, is not all that easy to do. In order to understand the astigmat, you just have to understand one certain thing—the Conoid of Sturm.

The Conoid of Sturm

Light that passes through a spherical lens is focused to a single point. Light that passes through spherical/cylindrical system (an astigmatic system) is not focused to a single point. It's focused to something that resembles a cone, but is different in very important ways. Because it looks like a cone, it is called a "conoid." The particular conoid that light forms after passing through an astigmatic system is called the Conoid of Sturm.

The easiest way to visualize a Conoid of Sturm is to make one for yourself. Go to your loose lens tray and pick up a +5.00 spherical lens and a +5.00 cylindrical lens. Now, bring them to a room with a slide projector and a screen. Turn on the slide projector and walk over to where the screen is. Hold the two lenses together in the path of the light so the axis of the cylindrical lens is horizontal (axis 180 degrees). What is the power of your little system? Along the axis of the cylindrical lens, there is a total of +5.00 D (+5.00 from the spherical lens and none from the cylindrical lens—remember that where a cylindrical lens' axis is, there's *no* power). Perpendicular to the axis of the cylindrical lens, there is a total of +10.00 D (+5.00 from the spherical lens and +5.00 D from the cylindrical one—perpendicular to a cylindrical lens' axis is where *all* the power is). For the next part, remember that m=1/d. The focal point for the part of the system with the +5.00 D of power is going to be 1/5 meter or 20 cm away from the lenses, and the focal point for the part of the system with the +10.00 D of power is going to be 1/10 m or 10 cm away.

Good, now what happens when we hold the 2 lenses in the path of the light from the slide projector 10 cm from the screen (Figure 4-8)? We see a perfectly focused horizontal line of light. What happens when we hold the 2 lenses 20 cm centimeters from the screen? We see a perfectly focused vertical line of light. What happens when we hold the two lenses 15 cm from the screen? We see a small circle of light. Any distance less than 15 cm, and we get a horizontal ellipse, and any distance greater than 15 cm, and we get a vertical ellipse. This whole thing: the 2 perpendicular lines, the circle, and all the endless ellipses when put together is called the Conoid of Sturm.

This, believe it or not, is what goes on inside your astigmatic patient's eye. Behind his cornea/lens apparatus, he projects light into a Conoid of

Figure 4-8. This whole thing, believe it or not, is the Conoid of Sturm. Light is not focused to a point anywhere. Instead it is focused into a series of ellipses and lines, and one circle.

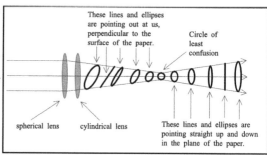

Sturm. What type of astigmatism your patient has depends upon where those 2 lines happen to fall. If both lines fall in front of the retina, the patient has compound myopic astigmatism. If the patient has both lines fall behind the retina, he has compound hyperopic astigmatism. If one line falls on the retina, he has simple myopic or simple hyperopic astigmatism, depending on where the other falls. If one line falls in front and the other behind the retina, he has mixed astigmatism.

What part of the conoid happens to intersect his retina will determine what the visual acuity will be. The smaller the cross-section of the conoid that intersects the retina, the less photoreceptors will lie in the "blur circle" (or blur ellipse, or blur line), and the better will be the visual acuity. Usually, one of the ellipses will intersect the retina. Sometimes, 1 of the 2 lines will intersect it. Once in a while, if he is lucky, the circle will intersect the retina, and in this instance, his visual acuity may actually be reasonably good. The circle is aptly named the *circle of least confusion* and if this is what intersects the retina, the patient will have the best potential for uncorrected visual acuity. When we refract an astigmat, we perform a 4-step process that is outlined in the following section. All we are doing during these 4 steps is manipulating the Conoid of Sturm to maximize the patient's visual acuity.

1. Maximizing the sphere—Placing the circle of least confusion on the retina.
2. Identifying the axis of the astigmatism—Finding the orientation of the Conoid of Sturm.
3. Negating the power of the astigmatism—Collapsing the Conoid of Sturm to a single point.
4. Refining the sphere—Placing the resulting point on the retina.

Maximizing the Sphere

Maximizing the sphere of the astigmat is not significantly different than refracting the spherical myope or spherical hyperope. The goals of all these are the same—to focus parallel light to the smallest possible shape onto the retina, and thereby maximize visual acuity. In the case of spherical myopes

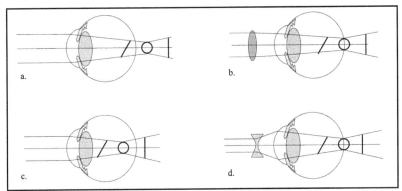

Figure 4-9. If the Conoid of Sturm is situated so that the circle of least confusion is located behind the retina (a), a plus lens can be used to move the conoid forward so that the circle is on the retina (b). If the Conoid of Sturm is situated so that the circle of least confusion is located in front of the retina (c), a minus lens can be used to move the conoid back so that the circle is on the retina (d).

and spherical hyperopes, the smallest shape is, as described above, a single point.

For the astigmat, it is impossible to bring a single point onto the retina merely by manipulation with spherical lenses. This is so because the light is not focused to a single point anywhere. Rather, as explained above, it is focused to lines, ellipses, and circles. Although we cannot change the shape of any Conoid of Sturm with spherical lenses, we can change its position within the eye with them. Even though we can't bring a single point of light to lie on the retina, we will still change visual acuity if we bring different parts of the conoid onto the retina. Remember that the bigger the cross-section of the Conoid of Sturm that intersects the retina, the worse the visual acuity. The smallest part of any Conoid of Sturm is the circle of least confusion and, therefore, visual acuity will be maximized when the circle of least confusion is brought to lie directly on the retina.

Moving the circle of least confusion to the retina can usually be accomplished with spherical lenses (Figure 4-9). If the Conoid of Sturm is situated in such a way that the circle of least confusion is located anterior to the retina, up in the vitreous, minus lenses should be placed in front of the cornea to push the image back until it sits atop the retina. This technique is really no different than that used in refracting the spherical myope that is described above. Likewise, if the conoid is situated so that the circle of least confusion is located posterior to the retina, plus lenses should be placed in front of the cornea to bring the image forward until it sits on the retina. The technique here is no different than that used in refracting the spherical hyperope as described above.

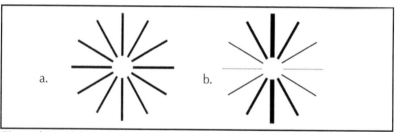

Figure 4-10. (a) How the daisy wheel looks to a patient without astigmatism. (b) How the daisy wheel may look to a patient with with-the-rule astigmatism.

Bringing an astigmat's circle of least confusion onto the retina is the first step taken in refracting every astigmat. This step is called *maximizing the sphere* and is performed entirely with spherical lenses. The endpoint of this part of the refraction occurs when you can't improve on the visual acuity any more with spherical lenses. For patients with just a little bit of astigmatism, this may be 20/20 minus or 20/25; and for patients with a lot of astigmatism, it may be 20/100 or worse. In either case, you know that when you can no longer improve on the visual acuity with spherical lenses, the circle of least confusion must be lying on the retina. At this point, it is time to change the shape of the Conoid of Sturm, rather than just the position. What we actually want to do is to collapse the conoid to a single point, a miraculous feat that is achieved through the use of cylindrical lenses.

Every cylindrical lens is defined by its axis and power. Therefore it makes sense that treating a patient's astigmatism must be a 2-step process. In the first step, you need to figure out the axis of the astigmatism that your patient has. This step is important because it really tells you how the Conoid of Sturm is sitting in his eye—which direction those 2 lines are pointing in. The second step involves negating the power of the patient's astigmatism, and here, you collapse the conoid to a single point. It is important that these 2 steps are carried out in that specific order. The axis of the astigmatism *must* be identified before any attempt is made to negate the power.

Identifying the Axis of the Astigmatism

There are a few ways you can identify the axis of your patient's astigmatism, and I will go over three of them, the *daisy wheel, stenopeic slit,* and *Jackson cross cylinder.*

Daisy Wheel

The daisy wheel (Figure 4-10) is included it here for the sake of completeness, but it is not the something that gets used on a daily basis. The daisy wheel is a circle made up of (usually) 12 radial lines. It is projected in the exam lane much the way the Snellen chart is, and the patient is asked to look

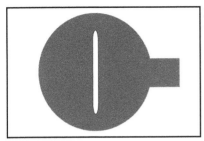

Figure 4-11. The stenopeic slit is a device that may be fit into trial frames. It is a useful tool to find the axis of a patient's astigmatism.

at it from 20 feet away. If a patient without astigmatism, be he emmetrope or ametrope, looks at the daisy wheel, all the radial lines will look alike. If he is an emmetrope, they will all appear equally sharp, and if he is an ametrope, they will all look equally blurry.

However, if a patient with astigmatism looks at the daisy wheel, one of the radial lines will appear brighter and sharper than the others. Which line looks sharpest will depend upon the particular Conoid of Sturm that the patient has inside of his eye, and where that conoid happens to be sitting. The key to the daisy wheel depends upon the fact that each Conoid of Sturm has those 2 lines where light can be focused. When one of those lines is closer to the retina than the other, one axis of the daisy wheel will be sharper, while the axis perpendicular to it will be much less sharp. You now know (within 15 degrees or so) the axis of your patient's astigmatism.

Stenopeic Slit

Another method to find the axis of a patient's astigmatism relies on a special piece of equipment called the stenopeic slit (Figure 4-11). This device, which looks like an occluder with a 1 to 2 mm slit cut into it, can usually be found in your set of trial lenses, and is meant to be used in trial frames. Basically this is an elongated pinhole. The pinhole, remember, blocks almost all light hitting the cornea, allowing only perpendicular light to enter, and thus circumvents the patient's light-bending system. The stenopeic slit works in a similar way, but it lets a whole line of light through instead of just a point. When a patient with astigmatism looks through the stenopeic slit, the image will appear sharpest when the line is turned in such a way that it lines up with 1 of the 2 lines of the Conoid of Sturm.

Here's where your patient can help you. Have him put on the trial frames with the stenopeic slit in place in front of the eye being tested (remembering, of course, to occlude the other eye). Put up the 20/70 or 20/100 Snellen line for him to look at. Now, ask him to turn the knob on the trial frame that rotates the stenopeic slit, until he feels the image is in the sharpest focus. When he is done, the stenopeic slit should be lined up with one of the 2 lines of his Conoid of Sturm, and therefore represents his axis of astigmatism.

Figure 4-12. A hand-held 0.50 D Jackson cross cylinder. Note that the axes of the plus and minus cylinders are perpendicular.

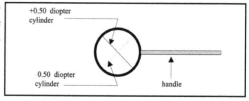

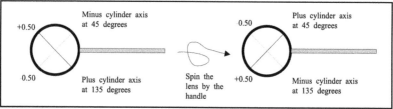

Figure 4-13. The orientation of the plus and minus cylinders of the Jackson cross cylinder can be reversed merely by spinning the lens by the handle.

The other line of his conoid, and therefore, his other axis of astigmatism, will be 90 degrees away from this first one.

Jackson Cross Cylinder

The Jackson cross cylinder is an unusual lens (Figure 4-12). It's actually two lenses in one. It's got a plus cylindrical lens of power +0.25, +0.50, or +1.00 with its axis pointing in one direction, and a minus cylindrical lens with the same power as the first one, but with its axis pointing exactly perpendicularly to the first one. The refraction of a 0.25 D Jackson cross cylinder held so one of the axes is at 105 degrees could be written as either +0.25 −0.50 × 105 or −0.25 +0.50 × 15. Turn the lens a few degrees, and you could write it +0.25 −0.50 × 90, and turn it a 90 degrees more, and you could write it +0.25 −0.50 × 180. Remember, the first 2 numbers in the prescription of any lens relate to the innate properties of the lens, but the third number only tells us how we are holding it (as discussed in Chapter 3). If this is not immediately apparent, you may wish to go back and review the cylindrical lens section of Chapter 3.

Another important thing to know about the Jackson cross cylinder is that it has a spherical equivalent of zero. That is, if you average the power of the entire lens, it comes out to zero. This is so because the plus cylinder and the minus cylinder, since they are of equal power and oriented perpendicularly to one another, cancel each other over the course of the entire lens.

The other powerful thing about the Jackson cross cylinder is that it can quickly be flipped around an axis. Say you're holding a +0.50 Jackson cross cylinder so that it can be written like this: +0.50 −1.00 × 90 (Figure 4-13). If you spin the lens properly, it can now be written as −0.50 +1.00 × 90.

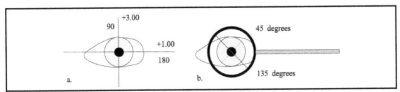

Figure 4-14. (a) This patient has astigmatism with axes at 90 degrees and 180 degrees. His refraction can be written as either +1.00 +2.00 × 180, or +3.00 −2.00 × 90. (b) When the Jackson cross cylinder is used to identify the axes of the astigmatism, the endpoint is reached when the axes of the Jackson cross cylinder exactly *straddle* the axes of the patient's conoid. In this example, it is when the axes of the Jackson cross cylinder are at 45 degrees and 135 degrees.

Or in other words, you've completely reversed the power of astigmatism in every place in the lens (except where it's plano, of course)—and all quickly and with very minimal effort.

We're sure that our patient has some astigmatism, and we just want to find out in which direction his Conoid of Sturm is pointing. Once we do that, we can try to get it to collapse to a point, but, of course, we can't collapse it until we know its orientation. When we hold a Jackson cross cylinder in front of our patient, and spin it as described above, he will be able to tell us when the axes of our Jackson cross cylinder are exactly *straddling* the axes of his Conoid of Sturm. If we hold a Jackson cross cylinder in such a way that its axes are straddling the axes of his conoid, then flip it, the patient should feel the image looks equally sharp before it is flipped as after (Figure 4-14). However, if we hold a Jackson cross cylinder in any orientation other than exactly straddling his conoid, an astigmat will see a change when the Jackson cross cylinder is flipped.

Now, try it on a patient. You've just finished the first step, maximizing the sphere, and have gotten him to 20/30 with a spherical correction. Next, give your patient something a little bigger to look at, say the 20/50 line, because the Jackson cross cylinder, with its plus and minus cylinders, can be a little distorting to look through. Hold the Jackson cross cylinder in front of your patient's eye. Ask him to concentrate on how things look (not to read the line, just to concentrate on how it looks), and then flip the lens and ask the patient to compare the two to see which is better. The easiest way to do this is to put down the lens and say, "Which do you like better, one...", wait a second, then flip the lens, "...or two?" Be sure to give your patient plenty of time with "one" before flipping the lens to "two."

If the patient feels "one" and "two" look equally clear the very first time, either you have found their correct axis, or there is no astigmatism. However, the chances are good that the patient will like "one" better than "two," or "two" better than "one." When either is the case, you must rotate (not flip) the lens to re-align the axes. To do this, you must first figure what was the orientation of the Jackson cross cylinder that he liked better (the "one" or the "two"). You then rotate the cylinder so that the axis you flipped around (the handle, if you will) gets rotated 15 degrees or so in the direction that the axis of the plus cylinder is lying in. This can be difficult to conceptualize without seeing someone do it. Basically, you turn the whole lens so that the handle of the cylinder rotates toward its plus cylinder. Practice with the hand-held Jackson cross cylinders first, because these have handles and are, therefore, a lot easier to keep track of than the ones in the phoropter.

You then repeat the process. Ask the patient, "Which is better, one...", wait a second, then flip the lens, "...or two?" If he says that they look the same, you are straddling the axis, this is the endpoint, and now you can go on to the next part. If he likes one better than the other, flip it back to the way he liked it better, and turn the lens so the handle rotates 10 to 15 degrees toward the axis of the plus cylinder. Then repeat the whole thing again. Keep repeating this process until the patient says the two look equally good (or equally bad, because the Jackson cross cylinder is a pretty distorting thing to look through), or you keep circling forward and back again around a specific point. Once the patient feels "one" and "two" look similarly sharp (or unsharp), you can assume the axes of the Jackson cross cylinder are straddling the axes of his Conoid of Sturm. Thus, you have successfully identified his conoid's orientation.

This step of identifying the axis of the astigmatism is an important one because the conoid cannot be collapsed without knowing its axes. However, regardless of how you found the axis of astigmatism, through the daisy wheel, stenopeic slit, or Jackson cross cylinder, you have not actually moved any blur circles, lines or ellipses. Therefore, your patient's visual acuity should be the same when you are done with this stage of the refraction as when you began it. Now that you have identified the axis of the astigmatism, let's use this information to finally collapse the Conoid of Sturm and improve on your patient's visual acuity.

Negating the Power of the Astigmatism

The best way to negate the power of the astigmatism is with the Jackson cross cylinder.

You have just used the Jackson cross cylinder to find the orientation of your patient's cylinder, so you know that the axes of the Jackson cross cylinder are straddling the axes of the Conoid of Sturm. In order to negate the power of the cylinder, however, you need the axes of the Jackson cross cylinder to line up with (not straddle) the axes of the conoid. To do this, merely rotate the Jackson cross cylinder 45 degrees in either direction (Figure 4-15). If you are using the phoropter, there will probably be a noticeable "click" when you get it into the proper position, but if you are using a hand-held one, you must find the proper position manually. Once you rotate the lens the 45 degrees, keep up that line that you know the patient can easily read (eg, the 20/50

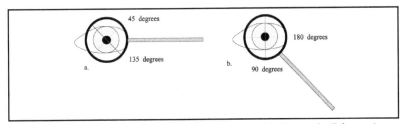

Figure 4-15. This patient (the same as the one pictured in Figure 4-14) has astigmatism with axes at 90 degrees and 180 degrees. His refraction can be written as either +1.00 +2.00 × 180 or +3.00 −2.00 × 90. (a) When the axes of astigmatism are found using the Jackson cross cylinder, the axes of the lens *straddle* the axes of the patient's astigmatism. (b) To begin to negate the power of the astigmatism, the Jackson cross cylinder must first be rotated 45 degrees so the axes of the lens now *line up* with the axes of the patient's astigmatism.

line) and ask, "Which is better, one?" wait a second, then flip the Jackson cross cylinder, "...or two?" If the patient truly has any astigmatism, he will like one better than the other. Flip the lens back to the one that is preferred. You know that where the positive axis of the Jackson cross cylinder is lying, he wants positive cylinder with the axis in that direction. Make sure that the cylinder of the phoropter is lined up with the cylinder of the Jackson cross cylinder (in modern phoropters this is usually automatic, but even so, may be exactly 90 degrees off), and dial in +0.25 D of cylinder. Then repeat the process.

You've just dialed in the +0.25 D of cylinder with the proper axis, so keep that 20/50 line up there and ask, "Which is better, one?" wait a second, then flip the lens, "...or two?" In all likelihood, he will still like one better than the other, should like the one with the white cylinder of the Jackson cross cylinder pointing in the same direction as the last time. If this is in fact the case, dial in another +0.25 D of cylinder (without changing the axis, of course). Every time you add 0.25 D of cylinder in front of the patient's cornea, you collapse his Conoid of Sturm a little bit within his eye. You bring the 2 lines a little closer together, and you make the circle of least confusion a little smaller. Thus, you will be improving the visual acuity, which the patient will start to notice after a while (although don't forget that the Jackson cross cylinder is a distorting thing to look through).

There is one more thing that you need to keep in mind here. Every time you add 0.25 D of cylinder, you are adding a lens with a spherical equivalent of 0.125 D [0.00 + (0.25 ÷ 2) = 0.125]. Therefore, you are adding plus power every time you add just a quarter diopter cylinder, the circle of least confusion keeps moving forward into the vitreous, and the visual acuity is potentially decreasing. Every time you add a quarter diopter of cylinder twice (for a total of a half a diopter of cylinder), you have added a spherical equivalent of exactly a quarter diopter [0.00 + (0.50 ÷ 2) = 0.25]. To compensate for this, merely subtract a quarter diopter of sphere from the spherical wheel of the phoropter every time you add 2 quarter diopter clicks on the cylinder wheel.

Keep that 20/50 line up there and ask again, "Which is better, one...", wait a second, then flip the lens, "...or two?" If he still likes it better with the positive axis lying in the same way, continue the process in the same way remembering to subtract a quarter diopter of sphere every time you add 2 quarter diopters of cylinder. If he feels they look the same, or likes it best with the positive axis pointing in the opposite way, you know you're done, and his Conoid of Sturm has been shrunken down to a single point. Now, you just want to make sure that the single point is lying on the retina.

Refining the Sphere

At this point we are relatively certain that our patient's Conoid of Sturm has been eradicated by the last 2 steps. If that's the case, and there's no other significant pathology (eg, diabetic retinopathy, cataract, glaucoma, ARMD), our patient should be reading the 20/15 line, or at least the 20/20 one. So we check. First, you need to take away the Jackson cross cylinder. Remember that the Jackson cross cylinder is a very distorting thing to look through, so your patient will naturally like things better after it has been taken away. Put up the 20/20 line and see how your patient does. If he struggles a little, and you are sure that the Conoid of Sturm has been diminished to a single point, it is likely that the point is not being focused directly onto the retina. We can use spherical lenses to move it about to get it there.

Dial in a couple clicks of plus sphere (remember to always get in the habit of erring on the plus side—it works against the patient's effort to try to help you by accommodating) and ask the patient if that looks better. If it does, you know you went in the right direction, and keep adding a little plus until he easily reads the 20/15 or 20/20 line. If the patient feels that things now look worse, you know you went the wrong way and you should dial in a little minus until he can easily read the 20/15 or 20/20 line. If he can't do better than 20/25 or 20/30, and you are pretty sure there's no other pathology to account for it, you probably haven't completely collapsed the Conoid of Sturm, and you should double check (axis and power) before you go on. Now it is time for end games.

END GAMES

End games are just little things you can do at the end of the refraction to make sure you have done everything right. These should always be undertaken whether your patient is an emmetrope, myope, hyperope, or astigmat. The easiest and most widely used end game is the red/green (or red/blue) test, and that's the only one that I'll go over here. The red/green test relies on a property known as chromatic aberration. If you've ever seen a rainbow

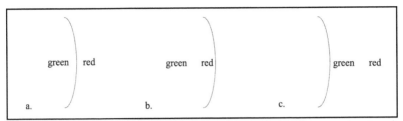

Figure 4-16. Green light is bent more by the eye's refractive apparatus than is red. (a) If a patient is properly refracted, green light will be focused in front of the retina the same amount as red light is focused behind it, and the 2 will look equally sharp. (b) If he or she is overplussed, the red light will be closer to the retina than the green and, therefore, look sharper. (c) If he or she is overminused, the green light will appear sharper because it will lie closer to the retina.

before, you're familiar with it. What this property states is that different colors of light are bent differently dependent upon their wavelength. If white light is focused to a single point on the retina, green light will be focused a little in front of it (in the vitreous), and red light will be focused an equal distance behind it (in the sclera) (Figure 4-16). Therefore, when asked to look at a red light and a green light, a patient will notice they will look equally sharp.

However, if white light is focused too far forward (in the vitreous), green light will be focused even farther forward into the vitreous, while red light will be focused pretty close to (if not right on) the retina. When asked which looks sharper, the patient will say, "The red." When this is the case, you should click in one click of minus sphere (to move everything back) and repeat the question.

If, on the other hand, white light is focused too far back (in the sclera), red light will be focused even farther back in the sclera, while green light will be focused close to (if not right on) the retina. When asked which looks sharper, the patient will say, "The green." When this is the case, you should click in one click of plus sphere (to move everything forward) and repeat the question. When the patient says that both look the same (and he should after just 1 or 2 final clicks), put up the 20/15 or 20/20 line again (in white) and make sure that he can still read at least as well as he could before.

There's a mnemonic to help you remember this. The phrase is "Go with plus." If the patient says the *green* looks sharper, he gives you the *green light* to give more plus, or, in effect, tells you to "go with plus." If he says the red looks better, you just have to remember to do the opposite and give minus.

Always be careful when a patient tells you he likes the red side better. To some people, in the dark, the red side will always stand out more than the green. Keep in mind that whenever you dial in a little bit of minus, the image will look smaller and darker, and some patients may misinterpret that as "better." You are at risk of over-minusing the patient here. If the patient says that he likes the red side better, you dial in some minus, and the red side is still preferred, you should probably just stop. Remember, end games are supposed to help things; don't let them throw off an otherwise good refraction.

VERTEX DISTANCE

One last thing you may have to measure in your patient is the *vertex distance*. The vertex distance is the distance from the patient's cornea to the lens. This distance is important in patients with high refractive errors—above -5.00 D for myopes, and +3.00 D for hyperopes. In these patients, the effective power of the lens will change as the vertex distance changes. Let's look at an example.

You measure a patient as a −8.00 D myope. The vertex distance during your measurement is 12 mm. Your patient goes out and buys glasses with a vertex distance of 18 mm. Believe it or not, if he has −8.00 D lenses placed into glasses at this vertex distance, they will work as if he were wearing −7.50 D lenses instead of −8.00 D ones, and he may only see 20/30 out of them.

When you do a refraction with trial frames, you will use a very simple instrument called a *vertex distometer* to measure vertex distance. This instrument looks like a small caliper. While your patient is wearing the trial frames, ask him to close his eyes. Gently place the flat end of the vertex distometer against his closed lid. Then open the caliper so the other end touches the back surface of the lens. Read the distance in millimeters off of the gauge.

When you are using a phoropter, there will usually be a small gauge that measures vertex distance built right into it. You may need to review your phoropter's user guide on how to do this, as some of these are not easy to find or use without specific instructions. As a general rule, do not use a vertex distometer when using a phoropter, as this will give you an incorrect value.

Once you've measured the vertex distance, be sure to then write it on the prescription that you hand the patient. Remember that you don't need to perform this extra step for patients with low refractive errors. For those with higher errors, merely write "v.d. 12 mm" somewhere on the prescription (there is often a specific space to write it) to clue the optician in to what the appropriate vertex distance was during the refraction. The optician will then manipulate the frames to ensure that they match that vertex distance, thus giving the patient the best vision possible.

Objective Refraction

The techniques described in the previous chapter dealt with the principles of the *subjective* refraction. All these techniques rely on having an awake and alert patient guide you in providing them with the proper lenses. What happens, though, if you have a patient whose mental status is such that he cannot answer your "better one, better twos" or whose vision is so bad that he can't read any of the lines on the Snellen chart? What do you do with the 2-year-old boy who not only can't tell you the names of the Allen figures, but barely sits still long enough for you to put different lenses in front of his eyes? These patients, who cannot help you to perform a *subjective* refraction on them, can almost always benefit from a good *objective* refraction.

In order to perform an objective refraction, you will need to learn how to use a device called the *streak retinoscope*. However, the retinoscope is not only good for patients with low levels of mental status and small children. Every patient who comes to you for a refraction will benefit from a good objective refraction. Without having to ask your patient any questions at all (except for, "can you see that light at the far end of the room?"), you can figure out a patient's refractive error down to within a half a diopter or so just with the retinoscope. Then you only need to perform a quick follow-up subjective refraction ("better one, better two?") to fine tune it. Because you are now making all the decisions instead of asking your patient to, you will save yourself a great deal of time with every refraction.

Copeland invented the streak retinoscope, and with it, he was a master of the objective refracting technique known as "estimation." Estimation is a way to estimate a patient's refraction without using lenses—just by using the retinoscope. With lenses being so available these days, it is a rare clinician who takes the time to learn the estimation technique. Most of us use the retinoscope in combination with lenses, utilizing a technique known as "neutralization." When I talk about "objective refraction" in this chapter, I will be talking about the "neutralization" technique.

Figure 5-1. The basic retinoscope. The light source is housed in the handle. The light emanates from the source as diverging light that then passes through a converging lens. The distance from the light source to the lens can be varied resulting in a change in the level of divergence or convergence of the light leaving the retinoscope. After passing through the lens, the light reflects off a semireflective mirror and leaves the head of the scope through an aperture. The examiner peers in through the eyehole that is located on the opposite side of the head from where the light emanates.

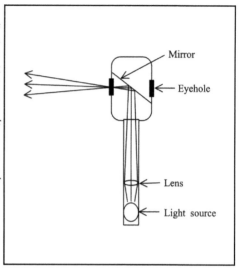

THE BASIC RETINOSCOPE

There are a number of different types of retinoscopes, but there are more similarities than differences in the equipment. I'm going to use *the basic retinoscope* in the forthcoming discussion to avoid a confusing discussion of the details of all the different types. The basic retinoscope (Figure 5-1) has a light source, a converging lens, a mirror, a place to look in, and a place for the light to be reflected out (180 degrees from where you look in). Overall it looks a lot like a long version of the direct ophthalmoscope, the basic difference is that the light leaves the scope as a linear streak rather than a circle—hence the name "streak" retinoscope. The ability to manipulate this streak of light is what makes the retinoscope so useful. By turning one control, the streak can be rotated around 360 degrees. Rotate it a little, and it lies horizontal. Rotate it a little more and it stands up vertical.

Then, by adjusting the distance between the mirror and the light filament, you can change the vergence of the light as it emanates from the retinoscope. Move the sleeve up (or down, depending on the type of scope you have), and the light leaves the retinoscope in a diverging fashion. Move it down (or up), and it leaves the scope as converging light. Leave the sleeve somewhere in the middle, and the light will leave the scope as parallel light. When performing the neutralization technique of objective refraction, you will always have the mirror positioned so that the light diverges as much as possible.

Pick up your retinoscope with one hand and turn on the light. Hold your other hand out so that the light shines onto it. Now raise and lower the sleeve, and look at the quality of the light on the palm of your free hand. You should notice that the light will be focused with the sleeve in one posi-

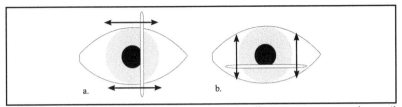

Figure 5-2. (a) When the streak is positioned vertically, it is swept across the pupil from side-to-side (as demonstrated by the arrows). When the streak is positioned horizontally, it is swept across the pupil in an up and down direction.

tion (up or down), and out of focus with the sleeve in the opposite position (down or up). When the light is focused, that means that it is converging (it has converged to a point on your hand). When you are performing objective refraction, you want the light to be diverging, so keep the sleeve in the position where the light is out of focus. Simply put, if the light is in focus on your hand with the sleeve up, refract with the sleeve down; if the light is in focus on your hand with the sleeve down, refract with the sleeve up. Whenever you pick up a retinoscope with which you are unfamiliar, you have to always double-check the vergence of the beam by performing this simple test.

Because of its name, you may think that the retinoscope is the ideal instrument for examining a patient's retina. This is not true; rather, the retinoscope allows you to examine a patient's refractive media or error by bouncing light off of his retina. The light that emanates from the retinoscope travels through the cornea, pupil and vitreous, bounces off the retina (fundus), and travels back through the vitreous, pupil, and cornea to pass through the retinoscope again and into your eye. This light is perceived by you as the patient's *red reflex*. It is in evaluating the nature of this red reflex that a clinician skilled in the art of retinoscopy can make both qualitative observations of a patient's refractive media (eg, cataract, corneal scars, irregular astigmatism), and quantitative measurements of his refractive error (myopia, hyperopia, and astigmatism).

When using a retinoscope, the light is never merely shined into the patient's eye and held steady. Information is gleaned from the red reflex only as the retinoscope streak is swept back and forth across the patient's pupil. The streak is always swept in the direction 90 degrees away from its orientation (Figure 5-2). That is, if the streak is standing up, it is swept side to side; if it is lying down, it is swept up and down.

QUALITATING THE REFRACTIVE MEDIA

The quality of the refractive media can be assessed by examining the nature of the retinoscope streak as it is swept back and forth across the pupil. Diffuse things like nuclear sclerotic cataracts and vitreous hemorrhages will diffusely scatter light on the way to and from the patient's retina. Both of these manifest as an overall dimming and diffusion of the retinoscope streak. Care must be taken when evaluating the streak in this way, however, as high refractive errors may affect the red reflex similarly.

Posterior subcapsular and cortical cataracts, and corneal scars are smaller and more sharply defined than are nuclear sclerotic cataracts and vitreous hemorrhages. These abnormalities will present as small, dark opacities within the retinoscope streak as it is swept from side to side. Because the red reflex is such a sensitive technique for demonstrating the presence of well-defined abnormalities within the anterior segment media (as discussed in Chapter 8), even very small abnormalities may easily be discovered. However, because it is based on the concept of retro-illumination, the red reflex is not a useful technique for determining the exact depth and location of the abnormality (also discussed in Chapter 8). Therefore, if you detect any abnormality in the ocular media through retinoscopy, it must be followed up with a careful slit lamp examination to determine its exact nature and location.

Irregular astigmatism is another entity that can be discovered through retinoscopy. When irregular astigmatism is not present, the retinoscope streak will remain single and straight while being swept back and forth across the pupil. However, when irregular astigmatism is present, it may cause changes in the shape and orientation of the streak. The most commonly recognized abnormal streak shape seen in patients with irregular astigmatism is called "scissoring." In these cases, the single streak is split, and the 2 halves form a "v," resembling the blades of a pair of scissors. Whenever the streak takes an abnormal shape, especially if it is split into 2 parts, the patient should be evaluated for the presence of irregular astigmatism.

QUANTITATING THE REFRACTIVE ERROR

The Importance of the Red Reflex

The refractive error can be quantitated by evaluating the quality of the retinoscope streak as it is swept back and forth across the pupil. This is probably the most valuable function of the retinoscope in the eye clinic, and, as mentioned previously, it is the basis for objective refraction. To understand how the retinoscope can function in this capacity, you first have to understand the nature of the red reflex as it leaves your patient's eye.

It is important to remember that parallel light that enters an emmetropic eye will be focused onto the retina as a single point. If you trace the ray diagram backwards, then, you will see that light reflected off a single point on an emmetropic retina will leave that eye as parallel light. Using similar logic, because converging light will be focused by a hyperope as a point on the retina, light reflected off the retina of an unaccommodating hyperope will leave the eye as diverging light. Because diverging light will be focused by a myope as a point on his retina, light reflected off his retina will leave the eye as converging light (Figure 5-3).

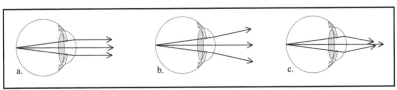

Figure 5-3. (a) Light originating from a single point on the retina of an emmetrope will leave the eye as parallel light. (b) Light originating from a single point on the retina of a hyperope will leave the eye as diverging light (remember that converging light that enters the eye is focused to a point on the retina). (c) Light originating from a single point on the retina of a myope will leave the eye as converging light.

When looking through the retinoscope, we can tell when light reflected off our patient's retina is converging, diverging or parallel. That's an enormously powerful ability. By knowing if the light is converging, diverging, or parallel, we immediately know whether our patient is myopic, hyperopic or emmetropic, and all without ever having to ask him if he can read the big "E" on the eye chart. By the nature of the red reflex, we can also tell if the light is diverging or converging a little bit or a whole lot. In this way, we can actually quantitate the amount of refractive error our patient has.

The information that the retinoscope gives us is where we sit in relation to our patient's far point. It tells us whether we are between a patient and his far point, right on his far point, or farther away from a patient than his far point. The far point is where a patient sees things in focus without accommodating. For an emmetrope, that far point is somewhere way out on the horizon (or clinically, 20 feet away). For hyperopes, his far point is actually somewhere past infinity, and therefore it can't even be clinically observed. For myopes, however, a specific far point exists closer than twenty feet away. For the −1.00 D myope, remember, this far point is 1 meter away. For the −2.00 D myope, it is 50 cm away (remember d=1/m), and so on (Figure 5-4).

So, how does the retinoscope tell us whether we are closer than a patient's far point or not? The key to finding this out comes from 2 features of the retinoscope: 1) the light emanates from the scope as a streak, and 2) we sweep the streak back and forth across the patient's pupil. When we sweep the streak across the pupil, we notice a couple of things. First of all, the streak is so long that we actually see part of it on the patient's lids, forehead and cheek. The second thing we notice is that, as we sweep the streak from side to side, the red reflex part of the streak may not move completely in sync with the part of the streak on the skin of the lids and face. The 2 parts of the streak will usually behave entirely separately, and that is the key to retinoscopy.

Sometimes, when the streak is moved from left to right, the red reflex may also move from left to right. This effect is called "with" motion, because the red reflex appears to move in the same direction, or *with*, the streak. This phenomenon occurs when the retinoscope is located between your patient and his far point (Figure 5-5).

Figure 5-4. (a) Because light leaving an emmetrope's eye is parallel, the far point is at infinity. For myopes, however, light leaves in a converging manner. (b) The far point for a −1.00 D myope is at 1 meter from his eye. (c) The far point for a −2.00 D myope is at 0.50 meter from his eye.

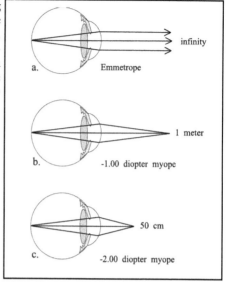

Figure 5-5. The retinoscope is held at 1 meter for each of 3 patients. Patient (a) is an emmetrope with a far point at infinity. Because the retinoscope is between the patient and the far point, the red reflex will show "with" motion. Patient (b) is a −1.00 D myope. Because the retinoscope is exactly on his far point, the red reflex will be neutralized. Patient (c) is a −2.00 D myope with a far point at 50 cm. Because the far point is between the patient and the retinoscope, the red reflex will show "against" motion.

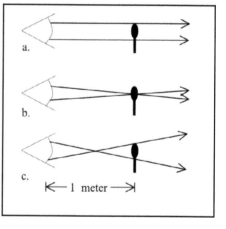

Other times, when the streak is moved from left to right, the red reflex in the pupil may actually move from right to left. This effect is called "against" motion, because the red reflex appears to move in the opposite direction, or *against*, the streak. You'll see against motion when the retinoscope is located farther away from your patient than his far point.

So, what happens when the retinoscope is located right at your patient's far point? Well, basically, you won't see any "with" and you won't see any "against" motion of the red reflex. Instead, when the streak approaches the pupil, the whole pupil will light up with red reflex at the same time, and stay lit up until the streak has passed completely over it and is onto the sclera of the other side. This is an important phenomenon to recognize because it will usually be the endpoint you're looking for when performing objective refraction. It is called "neutralization" of the red reflex.

Spherical Objective Refraction

So, how can we use this information to figure out a patient's refraction? Well, one way is to hold up the retinoscope, shine it in our patient's eye, and move our head back and forth, depending upon whether we see "with" or "against" motion, until the red reflex is neutralized and we know we're at our patient's far point. We can measure the distance away from him that we are in meters, find the reciprocal of that and we know his refractive error in diopters. That is actually one way that we can do it, but it is, of course, not all that accurate. In addition, it would only work for myopes because there is no way we could ever get far enough away from an emmetrope or hyperope to be at his far point (an emmetrope's far point is at infinity, and a hyperope's is even farther than infinity—which is, of course, impossible). A better way to do it is for us to stay still, keep the retinoscope at a certain, known distance, and move the patient's far point back and forth around us.

Let's look at some examples—first let's look at an emmetrope. Normally, his far point will be at infinity. However, if we hold up a +1.50 D lens, we artificially make him a -1.50 myope, and his far point is suddenly at 2/3 meter (Figure 5-6). Take a +2.50 hyperope. Normally his far point will be located in some impossible place beyond infinity. Hold up a +4.00 D lens, and we suddenly turn him into a -1.50 myope with a far point at 2/3 meter. Lastly, take a -2.50 myope. Hold up a -1.00 D lens, we change him into a -1.50 myope with a far point at 2/3 meter. See how much easier it is moving a patient's far point around than it is to move the retinoscope (and us with it)?

The 2/3 meter distance is an important one, and that's why I used it for all three examples above. This 2/3 meter, or 66 cm, or 1.50 D is known as the *working distance*. It's called that because when you retinoscope properly, the retinoscope is positioned about arm's distance away from your patient, and arm's distance works out to about 66 cm for most clinicians. Therefore, you too should get in the habit of being arm's distance from your patient when performing retinoscopy, and holding that scope 66 cm away from your patient's eye. One of the biggest mistakes most new retinoscopists make is that they get in too close to get a better view of the red reflex, and perform their retinoscopy from 40 or 50 cm away instead of 66. It's the difference between needing to hold up a +1.50 D lens to be at an emmetrope's far point and a +2.50 D lens, so please make sure you keep your working distance at the full 66 cm.

We've established that the *direction* of the red reflex will change as you move your patient's far point back and forth around your retinoscope. If the far point is behind you, you'll see "with" motion through the retinoscope, and

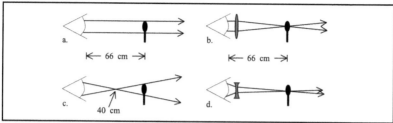

Figure 5-6. The typical working distance for retinoscopy is 66 cm. Lenses can be held in front of a patient's eye to move his far point to that distance. (a) An emmetrope has a far point at infinity. Because the retinoscope is between the patient and his or her far point, the observer sees "with" motion. (b) If a +1.50 lens is placed in front of the patient's eye, the far pint is brought up to 66 cm, and the red reflex is neutralized. (c) A –2.50 myope has a far point at 40 cm. Because the far point is between the patient and the retinoscope, the observer sees "against" motion. (d) If a –1.00 lens is placed in front of the patient's eye, the far point is moved back to 66 cm and the red reflex is neutralized.

if it's in front of you, you'll see "against" motion. What you need to recognize next is how the quality of the red reflex changes as you move your patient's far point around. When the far point is a great distance away from your retinoscope (whether in front or behind), the red reflex streak will be narrow and will appear to move across the pupil slowly when compared to the part of the streak that falls on the face. As the far point is manipulated with lenses and comes closer and closer to the retinoscope, the red reflex will appear wider and faster until it is so wide and fast that the whole pupil just fills with light and the red reflex is neutralized. At the point of neutralization, as discussed above, the retinoscope will be sitting exactly on your patient's far point, and you'll have reached your endpoint.

That is all there really is to know about spherical objective refraction. By observing your patient's red reflex's directionality ("with" vs "against" motion) and quality (thin and slow vs fat and fast), you can manipulate his far point with lenses to place it exactly where you're holding the retinoscope—namely 66 cm (or 1.50 D) away. Let's look at an example (Figure 5-7).

Sit a patient down and ask him to keep both eyes open and look past you at a light 20 feet away (we want to make sure he is not accommodating). Turn the lights way down in the room to help you see the streak and the reflex. You're going to look at his right eye first so hold the retinoscope in your right hand, look through it with your right eye, and place your left hand on his right shoulder. You want to keep your left elbow straight to ensure that the retinoscope is 66 cm away from your patient's eye. Sweep the streak back and forth and notice that you'll get a thin, slow streak that has 'against' movement. By the streak's directionality ("against" motion), you know the patient's far point is in front of you, somewhere between your patient's eye and your retinoscope. By knowing the streak's quality (thin and slow), you know it is

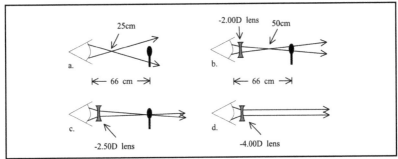

Figure 5-7. (a) A –4.00 D myope has a near point at 25 cm. Because we retinoscope with a working distance of 66 cm, his or her near point falls between his eye and the retinoscope and we see "against" motion with a thin, slow quality. (b) When we put up a –2.00 D lens, we move his or her far point out to 50 cm. We still see "against" motion, but it is fatter and faster. (c) When we put up a –2.50 lens, we bring his far point to 66 cm and the red reflex is neutralized. (d) We want him to see well at infinity, so we subtract the 1.50 D accounting for the 2/3 meter working distance and give an Rx of –4.00 D.

a great distance in front of you. You want to move the far point back toward you, so put up a pretty strong minus lens—say, a –2.00 D lens. Now you still see 'against' movement, but the streak is very wide and fast. By observing the change in the quality of the streak, you know you've moved things in the right direction, but the far point is still in front of you (because it is still "against"). Put down the –2.00 D lens and hold up a –2.50 lens. At this point you will see total neutralization, so you know that with a –2.50 lens his far point is at 66 cm (or 2/3 meter or 1.50 D) because that's how far away the retinoscope is.

Now you don't give him the –2.50 in his new eyeglasses because this would only allow him to see things in focus if they were exactly 66 cm away. To ensure that he will be able to drive in these glasses, you have to give him a far point on the horizon, not at 66 cm. To do this, mathematically subtract that 1.50 D that brought his far point to 66 cm. So instead of giving a prescription for –2.50 D, you give a prescription for –4.00 D (–4.00=–2.50 –1.50). In that way, his far point will be at infinity. It is time for his second eye.

Now you have to do the left eye, so hold the retinoscope in your left hand, look through it with your left eye, and put your right hand on his left shoulder, keeping your elbow straight to ensure your working distance of 66 cm. Look through the retinoscope, sweep the streak from side to side, and notice that you get a fairly wide, fairly fast streak that has 'with' motion. Take a good guess and put up a +1.50 lens. When you sweep now, you notice that the red reflex is neutralized. So do you give him the +1.50? No, of course not. If you gave him the +1.50, he'd be able to see everything in perfect focus at 66 cm away, but that's not why he came to us. He wants to see things on the horizon in focus. So, you subtract out the +1.50 for the working distance, and he should see great with plano.

There's an important point to remember here. If your working distance is 66 cm, you end up adding +1.50 D to everybody's prescription to neutralize their red reflex. To get their eyeglasses prescription, you can't forget to subtract that 1.50 D. It sounds easy now, but just don't forget in the heat of the moment in the eye clinic. And that's really all there is to it for spherical objective refraction.

Astigmatic Objective Refraction

Performing objective refraction on someone with astigmatism is not all that much harder than on someone without it. You just have to do everything twice and always remember where you are. With spherical patients, there were a few qualities about the red reflex you had to learn to recognize. You had to know the directionality (with vs against motion), and the quality (thin and slow vs fat and fast). With astigmats, there is one other thing you have to look for, and it's called *break*. Break occurs when the part of the streak that falls on the face does not line up with the part of the streak that's the red reflex (Figure 5-8). When you see a break in the streak like that, you can be sure of two things: 1) that your patient has astigmatism, and 2) that the streak is not currently lined up with one of the axes of his astigmatism.

Identifying the Axis of the Astigmatism.

The first thing to do when you see a break in the red reflex is to keep moving the streak back and forth across the pupil, and at the same time, rotate the mirror in the retinoscope handle. By doing this, you will cause the retinoscope streak to rotate as well. When you rotate the streak in one direction, you may notice the break actually seems to get worse, while if you rotate it in the other direction, the break will actually get less and less. Keep rotating in the direction that gives you less and less break until eventually the break will disappear. At this point, the streak is lying along one of the axes of your patient's astigmatism (Figure 5-8).

Check your work. You know that your patient has 2 axes of astigmatism, and you know the second axis is 90 degrees away (in either direction). Quickly rotate the streak 90 degrees in either direction and sweep it back and forth across the pupil. You should not see any break here either. If you do, either you have to refine things a little bit, or your patient's astigmatism is irregular.

Finding the Power of the Astigmatism

Now that you have found the 2 axes of your patient's astigmatism, it is time to find the power. There are 2 ways you can do this that both accomplish the same thing and just represent 2 different ways of conceptualizing

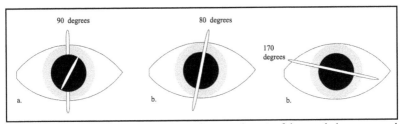

Figure 5-8. (a) The streak has a break in it because the axis of the streak does not equal 1 of the 2 axes of the patient's astigmatism. (b) When the retinoscope streak is rotated so that it lies along 1 of the astigmatic axes, the break in the streak will disappear. (c) The second axis of astigmatism lies exactly 90 degrees away from the first one. No break should be seen in the streak here either.

astigmatism. The first way is performed with just spherical lenses, and the second uses spherical and cylindrical ones.

Here is how to do it with just spherical lenses. You know you have a patient with astigmatism because you've entered a break as described above. You have found the 2 axes of astigmatism by rotating the streak until there is no observable break. Line up the streak along one of these axes and sweep the streak back and forth. Manipulate the far-point along this axis with lenses just like you did for your spherical patients until you put up the right lens to observe neutralization of the red reflex. Subtract the diopteric value of your working distance (1.50 D for a working distance of 66 cm remember), and you have the refractive power of the cylinder whose axis lies along the direction that the streak is pointing. This first step is essentially the same as neutralizing someone without astigmatism. Now, spin the mirror in the retinoscope 90 degrees and repeat the process. This will give you the power of the cylinder lying in the new direction. Put them together in a lens cross (as described in Chapter 3), and derive the prescription. Let's look at an example:

You scope your patient with a working distance of 66 cm and find that he has astigmatism, and that his axes of astigmatism are at 90 and 180 degrees. You rotate the mirror in the handle of the retinoscope so that the streak lies horizontally, and then sweep the streak in an up-and-down direction. By doing this, you get neutralization when holding up a +3.25 D lens. This means that one of his cylinders has an axis of 180 degrees (the direction the streak is pointing), and a power of +1.75 (in the direction in which the streak is swept). Remember that it's +1.75 D because we had to subtract our working distance (+3.25 − 1.50 = +1.75). Next, you rotate the mirror so that the streak is standing up and you sweep from side-to-side. When you do this, you get neutralization when holding up a +4.50 D lens. This means that this cylinder has an axis of 90 degrees (again, the direction the streak is pointing), and a power of +3.00 (in the direction in which the streak is swept). We can conceptualize that as a power cross where we have a power of +1.75 D at 90 degrees and +3.00 D at 180 degrees. When we do the math, we know the eyeglasses prescription is +1.75 +1.25 × 90. In minus cylinder, it's +3.00 −1.25 × 180. That's how you can refract someone with astigmatism using only spherical lenses. This is the best method for refracting small children who may not tolerate a phoropter or trial frames.

Here is how you do it with spherical and plus-cylindrical lenses (the technique used with a phoropter or trial frames). You have a patient with astigmatism, and you have found the 2 axes of astigmatism by rotating the streak until there is no observable break. Next you have to compare the quality of the streaks seen in the two axes, because you want to find the one that has either the most "against" or the least amount of "with" motion, and neutralize it with spherical lenses. If one axis has "with" and the other has "against," it's easy, just pick the one that has "against." If both axes show "against" motion, pick the one that has the *most* "against" (the thinner, slower one), and if both show "with" motion, pick the one with the *least* "with" (the fatter, faster one). When you've found the axis with the most "against" or least "with" motion, neutralize the red reflex with spherical lenses. Use trial frames or a phoropter because once you find the correct spherical lens, you'll have to leave it in front of your patient's eye when you go to neutralize the remaining astigmatism.

Now rotate the mirror in the handle of the retinoscope so the streak rotates 90 degrees. You should still see some "with" motion (if you see "against" motion, you did the wrong axis first, and you need to start over). Now, neutralize this "with" motion using cylindrical lenses. Hold the lens so that the axis of the cylinder lines up with the orientation of the streak—in this way, the streak corresponds to the axis of the cylinder, while the direction that the streak is swept lines up with the power of the cylinder. By putting up stronger and stronger cylindrical lenses, the quality of the streak should keep changing. If you still have "with" motion, you know you have to bring the far point in a little, so change to a stronger cylindrical lens. If you get a small amount of "against" motion, you know you have brought the far point in a little too far, so change to a weaker cylindrical lens. If you get a break in the red reflex, you know you've inadvertently turned either the lens or the streak of the ophthalmoscope, and you just need to turn them back again so that their axes line up with each other and with the patient's astigmatism. Once you've neutralized the red reflex in that axis, you are done. If you've kept up the original spherical lens, and have the proper cylindrical one, you will see that your patient's red reflex is neutralized in every axis. Prove to yourself that this is true by randomly rotating the mirror in the retinoscope in all directions and sweeping the streak across the pupil. All you have to do is write down what the lenses are that you're holding (subtracting the 1.50 D from the spherical lens for your working distance, of course), and you're all done. Let's do the same example we did before but with the spherical/plus-cylindrical lens method.

You scope your patient with a working distance of 66 cm and find that he has astigmatism, and that the axes of astigmatism are at 90 and 180 degrees.

You position the streak so it is standing up and sweep it side-to-side and get a fair amount of "with" motion. Then, rotate the mirror so the streak is lying down and sweep it up-and-down and still get with motion, but a lot less (the reflex is fatter and faster). Because you get less "with" motion with the streak lying down, start with it there and end up neutralizing it with a +3.25 D lens. Keep that lens up there (in the phoropter it's done automatically), and rotate the streak so that it's standing up. Sweep it from side to side and notice that we still get some "with" motion, but not as much as before in this axis. In front of the spherical lens, hold up a +0.75 D cylindrical lens and continue to sweep side-to-side. You will still get some "with" motion, but it is less (the streak is fatter and faster), so you know you are moving in the right direction. Take away the +0.75 D cylindrical lens and replace it with a +1.25 D one (keeping that +3.25 spherical lens right where it is), and find that the vertical axis is now neutralized. Check and find that the red reflex is neutralized in every axis—that's our endpoint. Look at our 2 lenses: a +3.25 sphere and a +1.25 cylinder with its axis at 90 degrees. Subtract the working distance (1.50 D) from the spherical lens and get an eyeglasses prescription of +1.75 +1.25 × 90.

Refracting in minus cylinder is the same as in plus cylinder, with a couple of things being just the opposite. With spherical lenses, first you want to neutralize in the axis that has either the most "with," or the least "against." Once you neutralize the sphere, you then leave that lens up there, and rotate the streak of the retinoscope 90 degrees. This axis should now still have some 'against' motion. Neutralize this axis using cylindrical lenses, subtract your working distance (1.50 D), and you're done.

All of these methods work to refract an astigmat objectively with a retinoscope. You will eventually find a method that you are most comfortable with. In general, when you refract small children with loose lenses, you will probably want to do it with just spherical lenses, because it's easier to chase a squirming, fidgeting child with a spherical lens than a cylindrical one. When you have someone behind the phoropter you will want to use both spherical and cylindrical lenses. If the phoropters in you clinic are of the plus-cylinder variety, you will use a plus-cylinder technique; if they are of the minus-cylinder variety, use the minus-cylinder technique. If you prefer trial frames, you can use either technique. Once you have performed an objective refraction, you just need to fine-tune it a little with a quick subjective refraction. It sounds like a lot of work, but you'll see soon enough how good a timesaver a good, objective refraction can be.

SAMPLE PROBLEMS WITH ANSWERS

Problems

1. With a working distance of 66 cm, we neutralize our patient's red reflex with a +3.25 D lens. What prescription do we give him?

2. With a working distance of 66 cm, we neutralize our patient's red reflex with a −2.75 D lens. What prescription do we give?

3. A colleague of yours is quite short. When performing retinoscopy, he must always use a working distance of 50 cm. He neutralizes his patient with a plano lens OD and +1.00 lens OS. What prescription should he give?

4. You perform objective refraction with a working distance of 66 cm on a patient who is a −1.00 myope in the right eye and a +0.50 hyperope in the left. What will be the lenses you will be holding up when you reach neutralization?

5. You perform an objective refraction with a working distance of 66 cm on a patient using only spherical lenses. When the streak lies along the 135-degree meridian, you neutralize the red reflex with a −1.00 D lens, and with the streak pointed at 45 degrees, you neutralize the red reflex with a +1.00 D lens. What is the eyeglasses prescription?

6. You perform an objective refraction with a working distance of 50 cm on a patient using only spherical lenses. With the streak pointed at 180 degrees, you neutralize the red reflex with a −2.00 D lens, and with the streak pointed at 90 degrees, you neutralize the red reflex with a +3.00 D lens. What is the eyeglasses prescription?

7. You perform an objective refraction with a working distance of 66 cm on a patient using spherical and plus-cylindrical lenses. With the streak pointed at 120 degrees, you neutralize the red reflex with a −2.50 D spherical lens, and with the streak pointed at 30 degrees, you neutralize the red reflex with a +1.00 D cylindrical lens. What is the eyeglasses prescription?

8. You perform an objective refraction with a working distance of 50 cm on a patient using spherical and plus-cylindrical lenses. With the streak pointed at 90 degrees, you neutralize the red reflex with a plano spherical lens, and with the streak pointed at 180 degrees, you neutralize the red reflex with a +2.00 D cylindrical lens. What is the eyeglasses prescription?

9. You refract a child with spherical and cylindrical lenses with a working distance of 66 cm. You neutralize him with a +3.00 spherical lens and a +1.00 cylindrical lens held so that the axis is at 180 degrees. Your attending physician wants to check your work but prefers to refract with only spherical lenses. You are in a hurry to go to lunch, so you hand her the 2 lenses she'll need to refract this child. What are the 2 lenses?

10. After spending a year at one clinic where you refracted with plus cylinder, you start working in a clinic where the phoropters are all in minus cylinder. With a working distance of 66 cm, you neutralize one axis (90 degrees) with a −2.00 D lens. To neutralize the 180 degree axis, you have to put up a −1.50 D cylindrical lens. What is the prescription you write in minus and plus cylinder?

Answers

1. +3.25 −1.50 (for working distance) = +1.75 D.
2. −2.75 −1.50 (for working distance) = −4.25 D.
3. OD: plano −2.00 (for working distance) = −2.00.
   OS: +1.00 −2.00 (for working distance) = −1.00.
4. OD: −1.00 +1.50 (for working distance) = +0.50.
   OS: +0.50 +1.50 (for working distance) = +2.00.
5. −2.50 +2.00 × 45 (or −0.50 −2.00 × 135)
6. −4.00 +5.00 × 90 (or +1.00 −5.00 × 180)
7. −4.00 +1.00 × 30
8. −2.00 +2.00 × 180
9. You hand her a +3.00 and +4.00 D lens.
10. Minus: −3.50 −1.50 × 180
    Plus: −5.00 +1.50 × 90

6

Near Refraction

ACCOMMODATION

As described previously, the relaxed eye is designed to focus parallel light to a single point on the retina. This is the case for all emmetropes and *corrected* ametropes, be they myopes, hyperopes, or astigmats. As also described previously, the relaxed, emmetropic, or corrected eye will focus converging light in front of the retina, and diverging light behind the retina. While converging light is something that the eye can only be exposed to artificially, the eye is exposed to diverging light all the time.

Remember that objects naturally reflect or emit light in a divergent nature. Thus, every time we stand close to any object, we will be exposed to divergent light. As we move farther and farther away from the object, light that has a large divergent angle will miss us, and we'll only be hit by light of a less and less divergent nature. Don't forget that it is not all the light that hits us that counts. It is only the light that hits our pupils that eventually gets seen, and our pupils are usually somewhere between 2 and 8 mm across. Eventually, when we're far enough away, only light that is parallel (or near-parallel) will hit our pupils, and all the divergent light will go right by them unnoticed (Figure 6-1). For practical purposes, this distance is 20 feet away, as discussed before; this is why our exam lanes are 20 feet long, and this is where the 20 comes from in 20/20, 20/40 and so on.

To focus diverging light properly, the emmetropic or corrected eye must expend energy in performing a function called *accommodation*. Accommodation is accomplished through changing the orientation of the crystalline lens/ciliary body apparatus. The cornea has nothing to do with it, nor does the retina. Think of the eye like a camera. The film in the back of the camera functions like the retina in the back of the eye. Conversely, the lens in the front of the camera functions like the cornea and lens in the front of the eye. Remember back to the days when cameras weren't self-focusing and you actually had to rotate the lenses to bring an image into focus? For

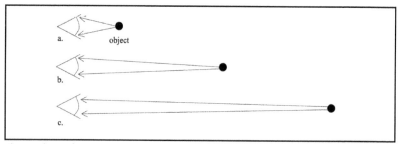

Figure 6-1. Objects emit and reflect light of a divergent nature. When the object is held close (a), the divergent light is still of a size and shape that it can be captured by the pupil. As the object is moved away from the viewer (b) and (c), the light that is captured by the pupil becomes less divergent until it is almost parallel.

the most part, all objects greater than a certain distance away (take 20 feet, for example) were in focus with the camera lens rotated all the way over to one side. However, as objects moved toward you within that 20 foot distance, you needed to quickly rotate the lenses to keep the object in focus. Without even realizing it, every time you rotated these lenses, you were simulating accommodation.

Accommodation in Emmetropes

When considering the emmetrope, you should also consider all corrected ametropes. It makes sense that the myope, hyperope, and astigmat who is wearing glasses should act much the same as the garden variety emmetrope. As you pursue your studies further, you will find that this is not exactly true for some specific cases. A monocular aphake, for example, may not tolerate spectacle correction because of anisometropia, even though he is 20/20 in each eye. Myopes can avoid reading glasses longer if they wear contact lenses, while hyperopes can avoid reading glasses if they wear spectacles, especially if they slide them down their noses a little bit. For the sake of this discussion, let's say that corrected ametropes act like emmetropes.

Like just about everything else that we do, accommodation is measured in diopters (Figure 6-2). This is fortunate, because it is a system with which we are already quite familiar. If an emmetrope wants to see something 10 meters away, he does not need to accommodate at all. However, if he wishes to see something at 1 meter away, he will need to accommodate. Figuring out how much he will need to accommodate is easy. We know that diopters=(1/meters); so if he wants to see something 1 meter away, he will have to accommodate 1 D [diopters=1/(1 meter)=1 D]. How about if that object is moved to 50 cm? Now the patient has to accommodate 2 D [diopters=1/(0.5 meters)=2 D]. And if it's moved to 25 cm away, he needs to accommodate 4 D. It's as straight forward as that. Figure 6-2 represents a way to write things out to help you keep things straight in your mind.

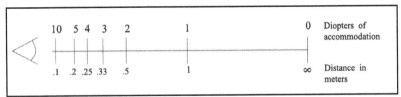

Figure 6-2. An inverse relationship exists between the accommodative power in diopters and the distance away the object is in meters. This diagram serves as a useful way of mapping out this relationship. In the clinic, the distance of 20 feet is used instead of infinity, thus saving thousands of dollars a year in heating and air conditioning costs.

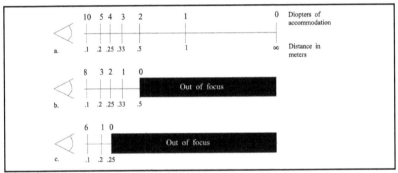

Figure 6-3. The accommodative diagram of a –2.00 myope (b) and –4.00 myope (c) are compared to that of an emmetrope (a). Past a certain distance, each myope has a range where everything is out of focus. As objects are brought closer, however, the myopes can bring them into focus with less accommodative effort. This ability increases with the level of myopia.

Accommodation in Myopes

Myopes have a head start on emmetropes when it comes to seeing at near. It is important to remember that myopia is called edness because myopes like to look at near objects that emit diverging light. An uncorrected –2.00 myope is able to see things that are placed exactly 50 cm away. Any object placed farther away than 50 cm will be out of focus, and if he wishes to see it, he will either have to put on glasses or squint. If he wants to see anything closer than that, he will have to accommodate.

If a –2.00 D myope wishes to see something held 33 cm away, he will need to accommodate 1 D (Figure 6-3). Why only 1 D when an emmetrope will have to accommodate 3 D to see the same thing held at the same distance? That's easy. Think of it that the –2.00 D myope is starting out with 2 D of near vision built right in. He needs a total of 3 D to see something at 33 cm away, so only 1 D needs to be added to the built-in 2 D in order to see it clearly. How much accommodation will he need if the object is moved to 20 cm away? The total of accommodation and myopia needed is 5 diopters [1/(1/5 meters)]; he has 2 D of myopia, so only 3 more of accommodation needs to be added. Two diopters of edness plus 3 D of accommodation equals 5 D of near vision.

Let's look at the −4.00 D myope now (Figure 6-3). He can't see anything greater than 25 cm away [1/(4 D) = 25 cm] without glasses or squinting. If something is held 20 cm away, he will need to accommodate 1 D to see it clearly. If the patient holds something 10 cm away, how much will he need to be accommodated? Well, an object at 10 cm needs a total of 10 D of accommodation plus myopia to be seen clearly. Our patient has 4 D of myopia, so he needs 6 D of accommodation to see the object clearly at that distance.

For those of you who prefer to memorize formulas here is one that may help:

(Diopters of Accommodation) = (Distance in diopters) + (Refractive error)

Let's look at the example in the last paragraph. We have a −4.00 myope, so we plug this into the formula as the "refractive error." The distance is 10 cm away, which is 1/10 of a meter. To change this over to diopters, we take the reciprocal of 1/10, and get 10 D. This is plugged into the formula as "distance in diopters." Diopters of accommodation = (10 D) + (−4 D) = 6 D.

Notice from the above examples that diopters and meters are not related in a linear fashion. That makes sense, of course, because of the relationship that "meters = 1/diopters." It's something that you should keep in mind, though, because it is very important clinically. To change your focal point from 20 feet away to only 1 meter away, a difference of about 17 feet, you only have to accommodate 1 diopter. To change your focal point from one meter away to 33 cm away, a difference of 2 feet, you have to accommodate an additional 2 diopters. To change your focal point from 33 cm away to 10 cm away, a distance of only about 9 inches, you have to accommodate 7 D more. So as you can see, the closer something is to your eye, the more you have to accommodate every time you move it incrementally closer.

Accommodation in Hyperopes

While uncorrected myopes have the luxury of accommodating less than emmetropes to see things held close to them, uncorrected hyperopes must accommodate more. Hyperopes, if you recall from Chapter 3, actually have to accommodate to see things at distance in focus, so when they want to see things up close, they have to accommodate even more. It can be tiring being far-sighted. Let's look at some examples.

A +3.00 D hyperope must accommodate 3 D to see something at 20 feet away in focus (Figure 6-4). If that object is moved to 50 cm away, he must accommodate another 2 D [diopters = 1/(0.5 meters) = 2 D], for a

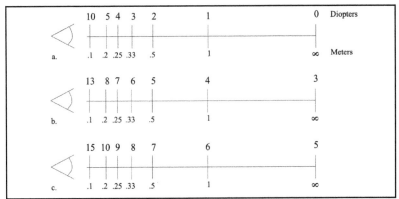

Figure 6-4. The accommodative diagrams of a +3.00 hyperope (b) and +5.00 hyperope (c) are compared to that of an emmetrope (a). The hyperopes must both accommodate to see things in focus everywhere, including at the horizon. At every location, the hyperopes must accommodate more than the emmetrope, and the +5.00 hyperope must accommodate more than the +3.00 hyperope.

total of 5 diopters, to see it in focus. If the same object is moved to 25 cm away, he must accommodate another 2 D for a grand total of 7 D. This can be a drag.

Similarly, a +5.00 D hyperope must accommodate 5 D to see something at 20 feet away in focus. If the object is moved to 50 cm away, he must accommodate an additional 2 D for a total of 7. If that object is moved so that it is placed 10 cm away, the person must accommodate a total of 15 D to see it. Table 6-1 compares how much accommodation 2 myopes, 2 hyperopes, and an emmetrope must perform in order to see objects at certain specified distances.

PRESBYOPIA

Presbyopia is the decreased ability to accommodate as one gets older. There currently is some debate as to the cause of presbyopia—while some feel that it represents stiffening of the lens with age, others feel it is simply due to increased size of the lens with age (remember that the lens continually grows throughout life). Regardless of the cause, however, just about everyone finds it more difficult to accommodate as they become older.

Young children can accommodate an incredible amount. In the first few years of life, most people can accommodate over 14 to 15 D. This comes in handy because most babies spend a lot of time looking at things placed about 3 or 4 inches away from their eyes. By the time most people are 70, they can't accommodate even 1 D. Somewhere between birth and age 70, everyone gradually loses the ability to accommodate. This loss of accommodation starts slowly, and increases steadily through middle age. A good thing

Table 6-1

ACCOMMODATION TABLE

DISTANCE	-4 MYOPE	-2 MYOPE	EMMETROPE	+3 HYPEROPE	+5 HYPEROPE
20 feet	Can't see it	Can't see it	None	3 D	5 D
1 meter	Can't see it	Can't see it	1 D	4 D	6 D
50 cm	Can't see it	None	2 D	5 D	7 D
25 cm	None	2 D	4 D	7 D	9 D
20 cm	1 D	3 D	5 D	8 D	10 D
10 cm	6 D	8 D	10 D	13 D	15 D

The amount of accommodation 5 different patients must use in order to see objects at 6 specific distances. Note that for each myope, there are distances where he cannot see the object regardless of whether he accommodates or not. Note also that each hyperope must accommodate at all times to see things in focus. At every distance, the myopes accommodate less than the hyperopes and emmetropes. See, being a myope isn't all that bad.

---

to remember is that most 44-year-olds have about 4 D of accommodation (it is easy to remember because it is all fours). As a general rule, the average 44-year-old has lost about 1 D of accommodation every 4 years since childhood. After age 44, he will lose 1 D of accommodation every 8 years or so until he is a few years over 70 and won't have any accommodation left at all. You can figure it out yourself, but the average 20-year-old will have somewhere between 10 and 12 D of accommodation left, while the average 68-year-old will have about 0.50 to 1.50 D left.

The big trick to presbyopia is that no one can comfortably use all of their accommodation over an extended period of time—most people can comfortably sustain only one-half of their accommodative potential. Therefore, although a 20-year-old emmetrope may have 10 D of total accommodation available, and can see an object placed at 10 cm away, he can't comfortably read text there for an extended period of time. He can only sustain accommodation of 5 D (half of the total 10 D that he has) and, therefore, can comfortably read text of significant length no closer than 20 cm away.

Emmetropes tend to become symptomatic when they're in their early-to-mid-40s. The average 44-year-old, remember, has about 4 D of accommodation available, and can only comfortably use half of that (2 D). Therefore, the 44-year-old emmetrope can hold text no closer 50 cm away if he wishes to read it comfortably. Fifty centimeters away is kind of far, but it is able to be done, and it explains why most 44-year-olds sitting in a dimly lit restaurant will hold their menus at arms distance. In my practice, I've found that the classic age for an emmetrope to get his first pair of reading glasses is 42 years old.

Hyperopes have a harder time, remember, than emmetropes. A +2.00 D hyperope has to accommodate 2 D just to see things at a distance in focus. A 36-year-old +2.00 D hyperope should have about 6 D of accommodation—of which he can use 3 comfortably. Two of these diopters are used just to see things at 20 feet away in focus. This leaves only 1 D of accommodation left to use on things held up close. This person will have to hold things at least 1 meter away to be able to read them—and he is only 36 years old! Needless to say, hyperopes in their late 30s and early 40s can be some of your more unhappy patients.

Myopes, on the other hand, have an easier time. Let's look at the 70-year-old –3.00 D myope. He really has no usable accommodation left in reserve. To see things 20 feet away, the patient will always need to wear glasses, but should be used to that because he has probably been in glasses for the last 60 years or so. To see things up close, he only needs to take the glasses off. With glasses off, everything 33 cm away automatically will pop right into focus. Granted, he can't see anything held much closer than 33 cm away, but that is a good working distance and should preclude him from ever needing reading glasses (assuming he doesn't mind taking off his distance glasses every time he wishes to read).

THE NEAR REFRACTION

The key to the near refraction is trying to figure out at which distances your patient needs to see things, and then giving him glasses so that he can see well at those distances. The near refraction is a very subjective experience for the patient, and is at least as much art as science for the clinician. There are 2 aspects to every near refraction that you must consider and of which you must make your patient aware. First, you need to know how easily your patient can read small print. More difficulty with small print reflects a need for a stronger reading lens. Second, you need to know the distance that your patient likes to hold things to comfortably read. This distance, called the *working distance*, is very important. You can give any patient a +10.00 reading lens that will enable him to read the smallest print in the dimmest of light. But will that patient be comfortable? Unless he likes to hold his reading material 10 cm from his eyes, the answer is certainly "no." The forces of "small print" and "reading distance" are constantly at battle. You must explain to every patient undergoing a near refraction that he will eventually have to make a choice between how small the print is that he wishes to read and how far away he wishes to hold the text. This becomes more meaningful when treating older patients, of course, with the advancement of presbyopia.

Children are normally easy to perform a near refraction on. Let's look at the typical 12-year-old male –2.00 D myope (Figure 6-5). Without correction, and without accommodating, he sees everything at 50 cm away in perfect focus. By accommodating (and remember, there is well over 10 D

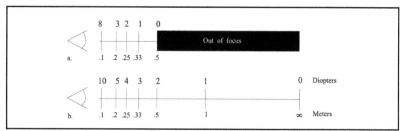

Figure 6-5. The accommodative diagrams of a 12-year-old –2.00 myope are displayed without (a) and with (b) distance correction (–2.00 sphere).

of potential accommodation), he can easily bring things into focus almost all the way to the tip of the nose. Uncorrected, though, his distance visual acuity will be about 20/80 or 20/100 or so. What happens when we correct with a –2.00 D lens? Well, the first thing the patient will notice is that his distance vision will sharpen, probably to 20/15. The second thing he will notice is that his near vision will not be compromised—he will still be able to see *everything* up to near the tip of his nose in focus. This is due to the fact that he still has so much accommodation.

Let's see what happens when our –2.00 D myope is now 44 years old. As we stated before, the average 44-year-old has about 4 D of total accommodation, of which he can use 2 D comfortably for a useful period of time. The patient presents with distance-only glasses and says, "When I have my glasses on, I have a difficult time reading. I can read if I take my glasses off, but I'm tired of doing that. What can you do to help me?"

When he gets a new pair of glasses, they will be *bifocal*, which means that each lens will be made up of 2 different lenses, one atop the other. The top lens will contain the distance correction, and when looked through, things on the horizon will be in focus. Because most of us tend to look down when we read, the bottom half of the lens is the ideal place to put the reading lens. The reading lens is defined by how much plus power we have to *add* to the distance lens to allow the patient to comfortably read. Because of this, the lens is called the "reading add," and we typically don't concern ourselves with the overall power of this lens, just with how much more powerful (or less powerful) it is than the distance lens.

An example will be useful here, so here it is. Let's say we have a moderately ed patient with a distance lens correction of –2.50 D. To help him read, we need to give a near lens that is 1.50 D stronger (more plus) than his distance lens. We don't say that we give him a distance power of –2.50 D and a near power of –1.00 D. Instead, we say that we are giving a distance power of –2.50, and a near add of +1.50. It's just understood that the "add" is "added" to the distance correction.

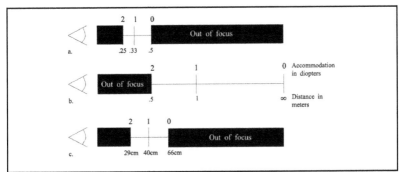

Figure 6-6. The accommodative diagrams for a 44-year-old –2.00 myope with 2.00 D of usable accommodation. In (a) he is uncorrected and can only see an object clearly if it is placed between 25 and 50 cm away. In (b) he is corrected for distance with a –2.00 lens. Now he can see everything clearly that is greater than 0.50 meter away. This in not acceptable for his job, so he is given a +1.50 reading add on top of his –2.00 distance correction as diagramed in (c). With this add, he can easily see everything placed between 29 and 66 cm away. Note the areas of overlap and that he can see all objects between 50 and 66 cm away with either lens. Note also that he cannot see anything placed closer than 29 cm away with either lens.

OK, let's go back to our 44-year-old –2.00 D myope (Figure 6-6). What we need to do is break down his visual functioning into ranges of where he needs to see, and provide a different corrective lens for each range. The first range is an easy one. He needs to see things at distance in focus. We refract for distance and find that he is still a –2.00 D myope. If we give that –2.00 D, the patient will be able to see everything at 20 feet away and greater in focus. He can then use accommodation to see closer things in focus. Remember, just because there isn't enough accommodation to see things at a comfortable reading distance in focus doesn't mean that what little accommodation he does have is totally useless. There are 2 D of usable accommodation left, so he can use this when looking through the –2.00 lens to see everything in focus from greater than 20 feet away all the way to 50 cm away. It ends there though. Through this lens, he will have a difficult time bringing anything closer than 50 cm away into focus.

Let's look at the second range, now. We ask the patient to hold a book at a comfortable distance for reading, and find that he likes to hold things about 40 cm away when reading. Forty centimeters away translates to 2.50 D of accommodation [1/(2/5 meter)=5/2 D=2.50 D]. It's tempting to give him a +2.50 reading add (the bottom lens of the bifocal), but this would make him unhappy for 2 reasons. First of all, because he would only be able to see in to 50 cm with the distance lens, and out to 40 cm with the near one, it would leave a 10 cm gap between the 2 where things would appear out of focus. Second, this person is young enough that he still likes to accommodate some to read; if you give a reading lens that corrects for reading distance completely (the 40 cm), he will have to hold things much closer (25 to 33 cm) if he accommodates a little when he reads. The patient will do much better with a +1.50 reading add. Give him a +1.50 add, and without accommodating, and he will be able to see things at 66 cm [1/(3/2 D)=2/3 meter] away. There are 2 D of usable accommodation left, which, when added to the +1.50 reading add equals a total of +3.50. When he accommodates these 2 D, things can be seen at 29 cm away [1/(3.5 D)=0.29 meters] in focus.

So let's put it all together for our 44-year-old –2.00 D myope (see Figure 6-6). Without glasses, everything at 50 cm away is in focus, and by accommodating, things can be brought into focus all the way up to 25 cm away, which is a relatively small range. If we give him distance-only glasses, everything from the horizon to 50 cm away will be in perfect focus; unfortunately, because of the person's need to read at work, this has become unacceptable. If we prescribe a pair of bifocals with –2.00 D correction for distance and +1.50 add for near, his problems should be solved. The distance lens brings everything from the horizon to 50 cm away into focus. The near lens brings everything from 29 cm to 66 cm into focus. Important things to notice are that he can see *everywhere* from 29 cm to the horizon in focus with these glasses, and that there is overlap between 50 cm and 66 cm away where the patient can see in focus using either lens. Our 44-year-old should be very happy with these glasses.

Time passes, and now our –2.00 D myope is 68 years old. At this point there is only 1 D of accommodation left, of which he can comfortably use only one half. He is currently wearing bifocals (–2.00 for distance with a +3.00 reading add) and says, "These glasses are great for seeing far away, and when I want to read up close, but I have the hardest time seeing items on the shelves when I go shopping, and I find it very difficult to see my computer screen." What he relates are common complaints of people as they get older (usually starting around age 50 to 52), and is representative of a major limitation to bifocals. The good news is that with a different type of lens, he can be helped.

Let's figure out his ranges (Figure 6-7). First he needs to see at distance, and according to his complaints, his current glasses seem to be doing a good enough job with that. You refract him and find that he is still a –2.00 D myope, and with that correction, he sees 20/20. He has essentially no usable accommodation left, so this lens isn't good for anything much closer than ten feet away or so.

Second, he needs to read up close. Again, according to his complaints, his current glasses are good. He still likes to read at about a foot away. His +3.00 reading add allows him to read at 33 cm away comfortably. This looks like it should be left alone also.

Now that he's older, he's developed a third range, called the intermediate range. Tasks that are performed at arm's reach—classically using a computer, playing piano, picking items off shelves—fall in that middle range that are too

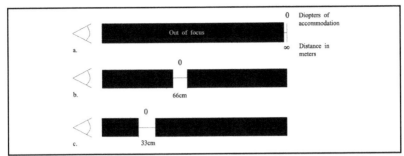

Figure 6-7. The accommodative diagrams for a 68-year-old –2.00 myope with no real usable accommodation. (a) Corrected for distance with a –2.00 lens, he or she can only see things clearly if they are essentially on the horizon. With a +1.50 intermediate add (b), he or she can see things held around 66 cm away. With a +3.00 reading add (c), he or she can read things held around 33 cm away. Note that things aren't in good focus unless they are held at 1 of these 3 distances.

far away for the reading add and too near for the distance lens. When he was 44, he had enough accommodation to see objects falling in that range through the distance lens. His accommodation allowed him a weaker reading lens (he was only in a +1.50 back then, remember) so he could also see this middle distance through either the distance or reading lens. Remember, with the glasses we gave him when he was 44 years old, he could see from 50 to 66 cm through either lens. Unfortunately, now that he has less accommodation, it's this middle range that gives him the most trouble.

What we have to do here is give him a third, intermediate lens. If you look at the lenses that he currently is wearing, you'll see that he has an area between 33 cm and 10 feet away where things are just out of focus. That third lens can be used to fill in part of that currently unusable range. A good estimate of what is needed for that intermediate range is half of what's needed for the reading lens. He likes +3.00 D add for the reading lens, so let's pick +1.50 add for the intermediate. If we give him a +1.50 intermediate add, this will bring things at 66 cm [1/(3/2 D)=2/3 meter] away into focus. That should make him happier. He needs to be counseled, however, that things from 33 to 66 cm and from 66 cm to 10 feet away may still be a little blurry (see Figure 6-7). That's just a factor of becoming older.

DIFFERENT TYPES OF BIFOCALS

Bifocals can often be difficult to get used to; patients should not expect to put on their first pair of bifocals and love them right away (although this can sometimes occur). There is definitely a learning curve associated with wearing bifocals, and patients should not get frustrated if it takes them a while to get used to them. They should especially be instructed that their "down" vision is going to be out of focus with the bifocals on. Therefore, they must get in the habit of tilting their head down when approaching stairs or curbs, allowing them to look down through the top half of their glasses.

There are many different types of bifocals in the market. For the sake of simplicity, they can be broken down to 2 major groups: "those with lines" and "those without lines." One very important rule to remember is that the bifocals they learn with are usually the bifocals they should stay with. It can be very difficult for a patient to learn on a pair of bifocals with lines, and after 10 years of successful bifocal wearing, switch to the no-line type. However, this can be successfully done in motivated patients.

Those With Lines

Bifocals with lines are the easiest ones for you and your patient to conceptualize. Basically, the top lens is used to correct distance vision and the bottom one is for near; separating the 2 is a visible line. The bottom lens is always spoken of as an *add*. As stated above, you should never describe it in terms of its actual power. Rather, just think of it in terms of how much needs to be *added* to the distance lens.

The biggest advantage of the bifocals with lines is that patients always know which lens they're looking through. If they want to see far away, they look above the line, and if they want to see close up, they look below it. Another advantage is that the reading part of the lens is fairly big—especially in a type of bifocals called *executive bifocals* where the line goes all of the way across the lens. This is important for patients who do a lot of reading, or who must see a large close area in focus at one time, such as the surface of a desk.

There are a few disadvantages to bifocals with lines. First of all, as any 36-year-old hyperope will tell you, they do make people look older. The biggest disadvantage, though, comes later when patients are in their 60s and have little to no accommodation left. These patients, as described above, will find they have a middle, intermediate zone where things are out of focus regardless of which lens they look through. It is these patients who need to make the jump to trifocals, which are similar to bifocals but have 3 lenses separated by 2 lines.

Those Without Lines

Bifocals without lines have a lot of optical advantages and disadvantages when compared to those with lines. However, you will find that the majority of patients will want them because they don't make them look as old as do bifocals with lines. Bifocals without lines are also called *progressive bifocals* because the power of the lens changes progressively from the distance correction at the top of the lens to the near correction at the bottom.

The main optical advantage of progressive lenses is that they do away with the need for trifocals down the line. Just by tilting her head, a female patient with progressive lenses can run the line of sight through an infinite array of tiny lenses of increasing power. If she looks through the top of the lens, there will be no near correction. If she tilts her head up a little, she may see through a +0.50 add, a little more and she'll see through a +1.00 add, a little more and she'll see through a +1.50 add, and even more and she'll see through a +2.00 add. In this way, even if she's 70 years old, she can use these glasses to see at distance, near, and all the intermediate distances in between without ever needing to change to trifocals.

The main disadvantage to using progressive lenses is that, although there is an infinite array of corrective lenses to look through, the part of the lens corresponding to a specific power may be quite small. If a patient needs to use the +2.25 add part of a lens, for instance, she may have to tilt or turn her head until she finds the proper part of the lens to look through. A lot of patients find that if they read with progressive lenses, they end up turning their heads more because they don't want to move their eyes behind their lenses and thus lose the "right spot" of the bifocals. Most patients find that the advantages of progressive no-line lenses outweigh the disadvantages, and will choose to stay with these more technologically advanced, and more expensive lenses.

A SHORTCUT ON ADD POWER

Now that you have read through this entire chapter, I'll give you the shortcut. Although many doctors don't like to admit it, most of us do develop presbyopia at the same rate as everyone else. We can use this to our advantage when fitting presbyopes with reading adds. Presbyopia represents a predictable 20-year slide from age 40 to 60. Most people under 40 need no add. At age 60, people plateau at about +3.00 D. A simple formula can be used to predict what add people will need between age 40 and 60:

$$\text{Reading add} = (\text{age} - 30)/10$$

Let's try an example. Using this formula, what reading add do we give a 45-year-old male? If we plug the age into the formula, we get: (45−30)/10=1.5. So we give him a +1.50. To a 52-year-old, we give a +2.25 D add because (52−30)/10=2.2 (which is rounded to +2.25). This is a simple formula, but it will work the overwhelming majority of the time.

SAMPLE PROBLEMS WITH ANSWERS

Problems

1. How much accommodation does a 30-year-old emmetrope need to perform to see an object at 1 meter away? How about if that object is moved to 20 cm away?

2. How much accommodation does a 20-year-old –1.00 D myope need to perform to see an object 25 cm away without his glasses on? How about if he puts his glasses on?

3. How much accommodation does a 25-year-old +3.00 D hyperope need to perform to see an object at 20 feet away in focus without his glasses on? How about if the object is then moved to 50 cm away?

4. Three 44-year-old men wish to view something placed 33 cm away. One is emmetropic, one is a –2.00 D myope, and one is a +3.00 D hyperope. None are wearing glasses. How much accommodation must each man perform to see the object? Who can see the object in focus? Who can comfortably read text at that distance?

5. Three 70-year-old women wish to view something placed 1 meter away. One is emmetropic, one is a –1.00 D myope, and the third is a +1.00 D hyperope. What strength glasses will each need to be able to see the object in focus?

6. Three emmetropes come to you for glasses. One is 15 years old, one is 44 years old, and the third is 70 years old. Each needs to view things comfortably at 20 feet, 66 cm and 40 cm away. What glasses would you prescribe for each of them?

7. A 15-year-old boy sustains trauma to his left eye that necessitates cataract removal with implantation of a standard single-vision posterior chamber lens implant. He is a –2.00 D myope in the right eye, and the surgery leaves him a –1.00 D myope in the left. What would you prescribe for glasses?

8. A 42-year-old woman comes to you with complaints of decreased distance vision. Although she doesn't wear prescription glasses, she is a dentist and wears safety glasses at work. Her biggest complaint is that she has trouble driving a car at night, but she notes that her vision isn't as sharp as it could be even in better lighted surroundings. You find that her distance visual acuity is 20/40 OU, her near is J1+ OU at 12 inches, and her MR finds her to be -1.00 sphere OU. She's interested in contact lenses. What would you do?

Answers

1. To see the object at 1 meter away, he will need to exert 1 D of accommodation because $1/1m = 1$ D. When the object is moved to 20 cm away, he will need to exert 5 D of accommodation because $1/(1/5m)=5$ D.

2. Without his glasses on, he starts with 1 D of myopia. He needs a total of 4 D of accommodation and myopia to see an object 25 cm away because $1/(1/4)$ m equals 4 D. Therefore, he needs to add 3 D of accommodation to his 1 D of myopia to see the object. If he puts

on his glasses, he loses that 1 D of myopia that he had, and therefore needs to accommodate the full 4 D.

3. This +3.00 D hyperope will need to exert 3 D of accommodation to see anything placed twenty feet away if he is not wearing his glasses. If the object is moved to 50 cm away, he will need to exert an additional 2 D, because 1/(1/2m)=2 D, for a total of 5 D.

4. The emmetrope must exert 3 D of accommodation because 1/(1/3m)=3 D. The myope starts out with 2 D of myopia, so he only needs to accommodate 1 D. The hyperope needs to exert 3 D of accommodation just to see things at the horizon in focus, and therefore needs to exert a total of 6 D to see any object placed a third of a meter away. Your garden-variety 44-year-old has 4 D of accommodation of which he can use 2 comfortably for extended periods of time. Because of this, both the myope and emmetrope can bring the object into focus, but only the myope can actually read text placed there for an extended period of time.

5. Let's assume that none of these 70-year-old women actually has any usable accommodation left. The –1.00 D myope can see things perfectly only when held at exactly 1 meter away, and therefore would not need any glasses to see the object. The emmetrope can only see things in focus when greater than 20 feet away, and she would need to use a +1.00 D lens to see the object. The hyperope can't actually see anything in focus without glasses. She will need to wear +1.00 to see at distance, and +2.00 to see the object at 1 meter away.

6. First, let's figure out the amount of accommodation needed to see at the three distances. To see at 20 feet away, no accommodation is needed. To see at 66 cm away, the patient will need to exert 1.50 D because 1/(2/3m)=3/2 D. To see at 40 cm away, the patient will need to exert 2.50 D because 1/(2/5m)=5/2 D. Let's look at the 15-year-old. Because he's emmetropic, he can see things 20 feet away in perfect focus. He has well over 10 D of accommodation on which to draw, so he can easily see any object placed at 66 and 40 cm away. He does not need to wear glasses. Now let's look at the 44-year-old. He can see everything 20 feet away in focus because he's emmetropic. He has a total of 4 D of accommodation of which he can comfortably use 2 D. By using this accommodation, he can bring anything into focus that is placed farther out than 50 cm, and therefore he doesn't need a lens to see the object placed at 66 cm away. He will need help, however, to see any object at 40 cm away. He is still young, and doesn't mind accommodating a little bit, so let's assume he won't mind accommodating 1 D to read up close. At 40 cm away, he needs a total of 2.50 D, so if he's willing to accommodate 1 D, he only needs to wear a +1.50 D reading lens. Thus, the 44-year-old can see at all three distances with the help of a +1.50 reading lens. Now let's look at the

70-year-old. He has no accommodation left. He can see at distance without glasses because he is emmetropic. To see at 66 cm he will need a +1.50 lens, and to see at 40 cm he will need a +2.50 lens. This man needs either trifocals with plano on top, +1.50 intermediate, and +2.50 reading, or progressive bifocals with plano on the top and a +2.50 reading add.

7. The distance part of his glasses prescription is easy. He shouldn't be symptomatic from just 1 D of anisometropia, so he should do well wearing a −2.00 OD and −1.00 OS. The reading part is trickier, though. He has his normal 12 to 15 D of accommodation in the right eye. However (and remember that accommodation is the job of the crystalline lens/ciliary body apparatus), he is pseudophakic in the left eye and therefore has *no* accommodation there. He is 15 years old and has a few years of schooling ahead, so we need to maximize his reading ability. He will need about 3.00 D of near help in the left lens—I'd give it to him as a progressive. His prescription would be: OD −2.00 sphere. OS –1.00 D sphere with +3.00 D progressive reading add.

8. This is a situation where you can do a lot to make a mildly unhappy patient very unhappy. She's a –1.00 D myope walking around with 20/40 vision only mildly symptomatic. If we give her contact lenses to correct her myopia, her distance vision should sharpen to 20/20 or better, and this should make her happy. Right? Probably wrong. Remember her profession—she's a dentist, a profession that is very dependent upon sharp near vision. If we give her minus correction, we will force her to work harder on her near tasks, and after a full day in her clinic, she may become fatigued. If she were younger, she probably wouldn't notice it. Likewise, if she was not a dentist, she probably wouldn't notice it. Unfortunately, she is 42 years old and very dependent upon her near vision for her livelihood, so we must proceed with caution. Fortunately, we have a few choices. First, do not give her anything and explain to her that you do not want to tip her into presbyopia with minus lenses and, therefore, she should continue as she is doing. Second, give her –1.00 glasses to wear when she needs them (when she's driving or at the movies, for example). Third (and I like this one best), give her contact lenses to sharpen her distance vision, but warn her of the onset of presbyopia. Since she wears safety glasses at work all the time anyway, prescribe safety glasses with +1.00 or +1.25 ground in. The lesson here is that you always have to be aware of your patient's vocational and avocational needs when prescribing glasses, especially in the early presbyopic years.

7

Motilities and Alignment

The fact that we are binocular organisms—that we have 2 eyes—gives us many advantages, but also makes things significantly more complex. Part of this complexity is the idea that the visual system works to the best of its potential if the two eyes work together. To accomplish this, they have to move exactly together. The other part of this complexity is the idea that, even if they move exactly together, what one eye sees is not exactly the same as what the other eye sees. Close one eye and hold your thumbs up so one thumb is in front of and completely blocking the other. Now, close that eye and open the other one. You should now be able to see that thumb that had just been hiding behind the first one. This happens because one eye is 2 to 3 inches to the side of the other and has a slightly different view of the world than the other one. Your brain has the difficult job of fusing these 2 worldviews into a single, understandable, 3-D image. We are evaluating this 3-D mapping system when we measure a patient's stereopsis (Chapter 1).

If everything is in working order, the 2 eyes move properly together, and the brain quietly glosses over the slight differences between them. If the 2 eyes don't track together, the patient has some sort of *strabismus*. To evaluate a patient's strabismus, we need to look at the *motility* (how the eyes move), and *alignment* (the position of the 2 eyes when they are not moving).

MOTILITIES

There are 6 muscles that move each eye in all directions (Figure 7-1). Horizontal movement is easiest to understand, as only one muscle is needed to move each eye from side to side. Each eye is moved temporally (toward the ear) by the lateral rectus muscle, and nasally (toward the nose) by the medial rectus muscle.

Unfortunately, things are more difficult when we move the eye up and down. This is so because the orbit, the bony, shot-glass shaped cavity in our skull that houses the eye and the muscles that move it, is not oriented straight

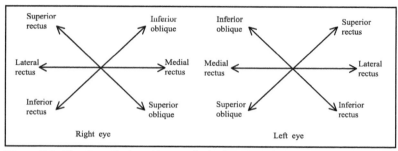

Figure 7-1. The 6 cardinal positions and which extraocular muscle is isolated when each eye is looking in each direction. These are the motilities of a patient who is looking at us.

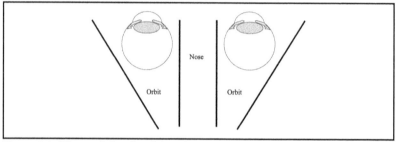

Figure 7-2. The medial walls of the orbits are parallel, pointing straight ahead. The lateral walls of the orbits are angled out roughly 45 degrees each.

ahead (Figure 7-2), even though our eyes are. Although the medial wall is pointing straight ahead, the lateral wall is pointed out temporally around 45 degrees. The advantages to this probably go back a long way. Animals that hunt like to have both eyes looking straight ahead to lock in on what they are hunting (think of the eyes of a tiger or a shark). Animals that are hunted, on the other hand, like to have their eyes looking off to the sides to make sure that they can see any hunters sneaking up on them from any direction (think of an antelope or flounder). Historically, humans have spent a fair amount of time as both hunters and hunted. It is possibly for this reason that our orbits are oriented in our skulls as a combination. Our medial walls are oriented straight ahead, like hunters, and our lateral walls point outward, like prey.

Because the lateral walls are not straight, if we only had one vertical muscle per eye, the eye would rotate when we tried to elevate it, making the world appear to spin. We solve this problem by having 2 muscles that work opposite each other to move each eye straight up and straight down. To look straight up, we call upon both the superior rectus and inferior oblique muscle of that eye to work together. To look straight down, we use the inferior rectus and superior oblique muscle.

When we test a patient's motilities, we always want to make sure that we are evaluating only 1 muscle at a time. This is easier for the horizontal muscles, because only 1 muscle is working to move the eye horizontally. If the right eye has a difficult time looking to the right, there must be a problem with the right lateral rectus muscle. However, things are more difficult when we evaluate vertical movements because, 2 muscles are working at the same time. Thus, if we know our patient's right eye cannot look up, we don't know if it is a problem with the superior rectus or inferior oblique muscle.

To properly test the function of all the muscles, it is important that we isolate each muscle individually when we test them. To do this, we evaluate the patient in what is called the *Six Cardinal Positions of Gaze* (Figure 7-1). It only makes sense that there are 6 cardinal positions because there are 6 extraocular muscles, and each cardinal position tests the function of a single muscle.

You'll notice that "straight up" and "straight down" are not part of the cardinal positions. This is because, as discussed above, each eye must use 2 different muscles when looking straight up or straight down, and we always want to test 1 muscle at a time. However, if you observe that your patient has difficulty looking up-and-out, you know the weakness must lie with the superior rectus. If he has difficulty looking up-and-in, it must be a problem with the inferior oblique.

To test a patient in the 6 cardinal positions of gaze, merely have him follow an object you are holding as you move it into all 6 positions. Most of us move the object so that it traces the letter "H"—right, up-and-right, down-and-right, right again, across the middle, left, up-and-left, down-and-left. Resist the temptation to trace a big square. Move the target slowly to ensure that your patient can follow it properly, and use an accommodative target (like the red cap on a bottle of dilating drops) rather than the bright glare of a flashlight. You'll find that as you move the object inferiorly, the patient's lids will naturally lower and obstruct your view. When this happens, just gently lift the lids with the fingers of your free hand.

When you are looking at both eyes at the same time, you are evaluating *versions*. If you are only evaluating the motilities of one eye, you are evaluating *ductions*.

If an eye doesn't move in a particular direction, the problem can be either passive or restrictive. If the problem is passive, it merely means that the muscle that normally would pull the eye in that direction is weak. If the problems is restrictive, on the other hand, the muscle may be fine, but the eye is stuck for some reason (eg, previous injury or surgery, thyroid disease). Depending on what your role is in the eye clinic, it may be your job to figure out if your patient's problem is passive or restrictive. The test to figure this out is the *forced duction* test, and it's just as the name implies.

To perform the forced duction test, first put in some numbing drops. Get 2 pairs of forceps with teeth, and let the patient know that you are going to use these forceps to try to move his eye. Warn him that he will feel something, but that it won't hurt, and that he may end up with a couple of small blood

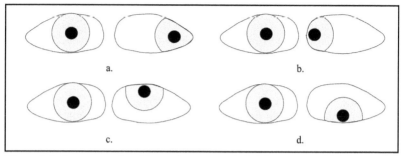

Figure 7-3. Four types of strabismus demonstrated: (a) left exotropia, (b) left esotropia, (c) left hypertropia, and (d) left hypertropia. In all cases, the patient is fixing with his right eye.

spots that will take a week or so to go away. Also tell him to relax his eye, and to let you just try to move his eye for him. Then, grasp a small amount of episcleral tissue just outside of the corneoscleral limbus with the forceps, and try to roll the eye into the position that the patient can't. If you can move the eye easily, then the problem must be passive – the muscle is weak. If eye doesn't move in that direction, there must be a restriction somewhere.

All this discussion dealt with describing eye movement. Next, we need to talk about the position of the eyes while they are still, their alignment.

ALIGNMENT

When we look straight ahead, our eyes are in what is called *primary position*. When most of us are in primary position, our 2 eyes are each pointing straight ahead, and thus each eye is locked onto whatever it is we are looking at. If we are doing it correctly, and each eye is in fact looking straight ahead, we are labeled *ortho*, meaning straight. If we are anything other than ortho, we have a *deviation*. What type of deviation someone may have is defined by two factors.

The first factor that defines a deviation is its direction (Figure 7-3). This is fairly straightforward (at least on paper). If the eye turns out (wall-eye), it is an *exo-* deviation. If it turns in (cross-eye), it is an *eso-* deviation. If it turns up, it is a *hyper-*, and if it turns down, it is a *hypo-* deviation.

The second factor that defines a deviation is how often it is there. If the deviation is there all the time, the patient has a *–tropia;* if the deviation is there spontaneously, but not all the time, the patient has an *intermittent –tropia*. In some patients, the deviation is only present when their ability to fuse is somehow disrupted. It may only show itself when one eye is closed or covered, when the patient looks into bright sunlight, is tired, has had of glasses of wine. These patients have a *–phoria*.

Table 7-1

ABBREVIATION SYSTEM FOR STRABISMUS

DIRECTION	PREFIX	ABBREVIATION
Straight	Ortho-	Ortho-
Eye turns in	Eso-	E-
Eye turns out	Exo-	X-
Eye turns up	Hyper-	H-
Eye turns down	Hypo-	Hypo-

TYPE OF DEVIATION	SUFFIX	ABBREVIATION
Always present with both eyes open	-tropia	-T
Sometimes present with both eyes open	Intermittent -tropia	-(T)
There only when unable to fuse	-phoria	-P (or nothing)

You will notice that the terms to describe the direction of the deviation (exo-, eso-, hyper-, hypo-) all have hyphens at the ends of the word, while the terms to describe the type (-tropia, intermittent -tropia, -phoria), all have hyphens at the beginnings of the word. To finish the job, all you have to do is combine the first half of the word (the direction) with the second half (the type), add which eye is responsible (left or right), and write down the combination to come up with the final description. For example, if someone's right eye turns in all the time, he has a right esotropia ("right" + "eso-" + "-tropia"). If someone has a left eye that points out much of the time, he has an intermittent left exotropia ("left" + "exo-" + "intermittent –tropia." If someone else has a right eye that drifts up only in bright sunlight or when he's tired, he has a right hyperphoria ("right" + "hyper-" + "-phoria").

It is commonly known that health care providers never like to write entire words if it can be helped, so fortunately, someone had the foresight to come up with an abbreviation system to describe these deviations in alignment (Table 7-1). Because the direction of the deviation is always the first half of the word, this is first half of the abbreviation as well.

Because the type of deviation is the second half of the word, it only makes sense that it is the second half of the abbreviation as well.

Now, just put the building blocks together. Our patient with a right esotropia described above is abbreviated RET. Our patient with an intermittent left exotropia is abbreviated LX(T). Our patient with a right hyperphoria is abbreviated either RHP or RH.

All of this discussion has been on patients with deviations when looking off in the distance. It is not unusual for someone's deviation to be different at near than it is at distance, and so the near deviation must be measured and recorded separately. To record the near deviation, merely add a prime sign (') to the end of the abbreviation. Thus, if a patient has a right esotropia at near, it is recorded as RET'. If he has a left intermittent exotropia at near, it is recorded as LX(T)'. And, the patient with a right hyperphoria at near is recorded as RHP', or RH'. If you are ortho at near, you are ortho'.

It is not uncommon for a patient who has strabismus to be more comfortable holding his head in one certain position. If the patient has a problem with a lateral or medial rectus muscle, he may adopt a *head turn* in the direction of the weak muscle. If he likes to walk around with his nose pointed toward his left ear, he has a "left head turn." If a patient has a problem with one of the muscles that moves the eye up or down, he may adopt a *head tilt*. If he naturally has his left ear drawn down toward his left shoulder, he has a "left head tilt." Often these head turns and tilts will give clues as to the types of deviations that patients may have. It is a good practice to ask patients with abnormal head positions to bring in old pictures of themselves to get clues as to how long they've had the strabismus.

If you have a patient with a head turn or tilt, it is imperative that you do not measure the deviation while he is in his abnormal head position. This may require constant reminding during the examination because he doesn't think his head position is abnormal; he is merely doing what is comfortable for him. Do not be afraid to gently move his head into a straight position with your hands if he is unable to figure out what you're trying to get him to do. You may have to do this a number of times during the exam.

You now should have a pretty good understanding of motilities and alignment in a qualitative sense. It's time to learn how to measure these deviations. To do this, we first need an understanding of the optics behind how a prism works.

PRISM

Prisms are a lot like lenses, but their surfaces are flat instead of curved. Because of this, they can't focus light to a point; they can only deflect it (Figure 7-4). If parallel light enters a prism, parallel light will exit it, just in a different direction. The light is always deflected toward the prism's *base* (the flat side), and away from its *apex* (the pointy end). Because of this, whenever we describe how we are holding a prism, we define it by where the base is. If a prism is held so that its base is down, as is seen in Figure 7-4, it is described as *base down*, which is abbreviated BD. If the base is facing toward the ceiling, it is *base up* (BU), toward the nose is *base in* (BI), and toward the ear is *base out* (BO).

It's important to note here that we don't describe the position as "base right" or "base left"—rather we describe it as "base in" or "base out." Therefore, when we hold a prism up, "base in" for the right eye will be opposite to "base in" for the left eye. We adopt this nomenclature because it makes more sense functionally, as you'll see when you start to work with patients with strabismus.

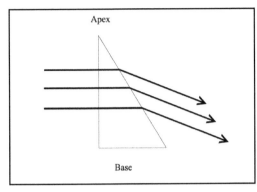

Figure 7-4. Light that passes through a prism is deflected toward its base. Note that when parallel light enters a prism, the light that exits is also parallel. The prism has no effect on the vergence.

How well a specific prism deflects light is dependent upon how it is held. A prism bends light most effectively when one face is perpendicular to the direction of the light. When using a prism on patients, the straight up-and-down side is typically positioned toward the patient, and the angled side is facing the examiner. Then, you merely have to make sure that the base is parallel to either the floor (when measuring BU and BD), or the wall (when measuring BI or BO).

What we are measuring when we use prism is the amount that light is deflected. The unit of measurement for this is the *prism diopter,* which is abbreviated $^\Delta$. The prism diopter is the distance that light has been deflected (measured in centimeters) when measured 1 meter away from the prism (Figure 7-5). Therefore, if you stand 1 meter from a prism and see that light has been deflected 4 cm, you know that you are dealing with a 4^Δ prism.

The significant shortcoming in the system used to measure the strength of prisms is that there is no room for negative numbers. I will grant that negative numbers are more difficult to work with than positive numbers. However, the trade off is that with prisms, because there are no negative numbers, you always have to remember the direction—BU, BD, BI, BO—in the back of your mind. When adding 2 numbers (4^Δ BU to 3^Δ BD, or 2^Δ BI to 5^Δ BO), you now have to remember if you're supposed to be adding these together or subtracting them to get your answer. If you were using a math system that had negative numbers, you wouldn't have to do anything extra here—the math would work itself out.

MEASURING THE DEVIATION

It's one thing to just tell a patient what type of deviation he may have, but we can't actually help him unless we measure it. Once we measure it, we can treat it, either by putting prism in his glasses or by fixing the deviation through surgery.

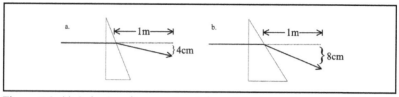

Figure 7-5. (a) A 4 prism diopter prism deflects light 4 cm when measured 1 meter away. (b) An 8 prism diopter prism deflects light 8 cm when measured 1 meter away.

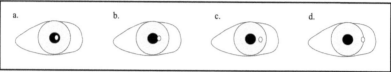

Figure 7-6. Estimating the deviation by the Hirschberg test. (a) is ortho because the light reflex is just nasal to the center of the pupil. (b) The light reflex is at the pupillary margin, and this represents a deviation of 30Δ. (c) When the light reflex falls half-way between the pupillary margin and the limbus, this represents a deviation of 60Δ. (d) The limbus represents a deviation of 90Δ.

Hirschberg Test

The Hirschberg test is a way to estimate someone's deviation just by look-ing at him. Specifically, we look at where the corneal light reflex lies in rela-tion to his pupil and corneoscleral limbus. To perform the Hirschberg test, hold a muscle light a few feet in front of your patient while asking him to fix-ate on a distant target (not the light). Then, look to see where the reflection from that light occurs on each eye (Figure 7-6). If the eye is straight (ortho), the light reflex should be just nasal to the middle of the pupil. If the light falls to the nasal side, the patient must be exo-, and if it falls on the temporal side, he must be eso-.

Next, we can get a rough measurement of how much of a deviation the patient has by evaluating exactly where the light reflex falls. Basically, every millimeter that the light reflex is away from the center of the pupil represents 15Δ of deviation. If the reflex falls at the pupillary margin, that represents a deviation of about 30Δ. If it falls between the iris and limbus, this repre-sents about 60Δ. The limbus represents 90Δ. Please bear in mind that the Hirschberg test is inexact, and should only be used to estimate a deviation.

Modified Krimsky Test

The Krimsky test is essentially the same as the Hirschberg test, except that we quantitate it better by using prism. When Krimsky first described his test, he placed a prism in front of the deviating eye, and used it to move the light reflex to the center of the pupil. The convention now is that we put the prism

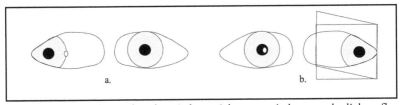

Figure 7-7. (a) We know that there is large right exotropia because the light reflex of the right eye falls on the nasal limbus. (b) We put a prism in front of the fixating left eye. The patient moves both eyes to the left to continue fixating with the left eye. Eventually, the right eye is moved into an ortho position that is recognized because the light reflex is in the middle of the pupil.

in front of the eye that is not deviating, the fixating eye. If the patient keeps fixation with that eye, he will move both eyes together when we put a prism in front of it, and eventually move the deviated eye into an ortho position. We recognize that this eye is now ortho because the light reflex falls in the middle of the pupil. Because we use this modified version of Krimsky's test, it is usually referred to as the *Modified Krimsky* test.

We set up this test similar to the Hirschberg test above. We hold a light a few feet in front of our patient, and ask him to fixate on a distant target. Then we look to see where the light reflex falls. If the light reflex falls somewhere other than immediately nasal to the center of the pupil, we know that the patient has a deviation. Up until this point, everything is identical to the Hirschberg test.

Pick up the prism that is predicted by the results of the Hirschberg test (Figure 7-7). Hold it in front of the fixating eye so that the apex of the prism points away from the direction that the other eye is deviated. In other words, if the right eye is exotropic (pointing toward the *right* ear), hold a prism in front of the left eye in a base in orientation (so the apex points toward the *left* ear). When this prism is in place, the patient will move his left eye toward his left in order to keep fixating on the target with this eye. Even though there is a deviation, both eyes will move together—when he moves his left eye toward the left, his right eye will shift to the left also. This will reduce, or even alleviate, the exo-deviation in that eye. If you picked up the correct prism, the light reflex should be near the center of the pupil and that is your endpoint. If not, put that prism down and try another one.

This test is more accurate than the Hirschberg test because it does use prism to try to quantify things. However, the endpoint is still a little fuzzy because we are relying on our ability to guess when the light reflex is in the center of the pupil. To get more exact results, it's time to put down the muscle light and pick up an occluder.

Cover-Uncover Test

The cover-uncover test is a good way to measure tropias and phorias in patients with alignment problems without motility problems. For this reason, it is a good test for measuring deviations in children. It is often not as useful for measuring deviations in an adult who has developed a strabismus later in life secondary to trauma, or an orbital problem such as thyroid disease. The cover-uncover test relies on the theory that when one eye is covered, the other one will want to look at the target. This is so even if that eye wasn't necessarily looking at the target before the other eye is covered.

To perform the cover-uncover test, have your patient look at a distant target like a letter on the eye chart. Then cover one of his or her eyes with an occluder while observing the other eye—if you cover the left eye, you will look at his or her right eye. Observe what the unoccluded eye does when the other eye is covered. If it doesn't do anything special, that means that this eye was looking at the target the whole time, and that eye has no deviation. If this happens, repeat the test with the other eye. However, if that eye shifted when the other one was occluded, we know that it had not been looking at the target when both eyes were open, and he must have a deviation. Because the deviation existed with both eyes open, it must be a –tropia. If the eye shifts temporally when the other is covered, it must have been too nasal, and, therefore, he has an esotropia. On the other hand, if it shifts nasally when the other is covered, it must have been too temporal, and, as a result, the patient has an exotropia. You can come to similar conclusions about hyper- and hypotropias.

You can now use a prism to measure what the deviation is. Once you figure out that your patient has a deviation, pick up a prism. If the deviation looks large, grab a high power prism; if it looks small, grab a small power one. Hold the prism so that the apex points toward the direction of the deviation, and hold the prism in front of the deviating eye at the same time that you put the occluder in front of the fixating one. If you don't see any deviation, you know that you picked up the correct strength prism. If you see movement in the same direction but less than before, you know that you picked up a prism that was too weak, and you should try again with a stronger one. If you see movement in the opposite direction as before, you know that you picked up a prism that was too strong, and should grab one that is weaker. The first half of the cover-uncover test is concluded once you have found the right prism.

Next, make observations about what happens when you uncover the eye that was just occluded. This time, look at the eye that was occluded, and make observations about its alignment when you take away the occluder. If you don't see any deviation here, then that eye is ortho. If you do see a deviation, you know that it occurred when the eye was covered, and it is therefore likely a –phoria rather than a –tropia. If the eye adjusts by moving temporally, it must be an esophoria, and if it adjusts by moving nasally, it must be an exophoria.

Measuring the deviation when you remove the occluder is similar to what you did before when you measured the eye when you put up the occluder. The major differences are that you put up the prism in front of the eye that is covered, and look at that eye when the occluder is removed. Otherwise it's the same thing. Point the apex of the prism toward the deviation, and keep putting up different size prisms until you are convinced that you picked one that the eye doesn't move behind when the occluder is removed.

It sounds simple, but don't be frustrated if you don't get it right the first time. Measuring someone's deviation with prism is one of the hardest things you will be asked to do in the eye clinic. One of the problems with measuring strabismus is that the deviation will often start to build as you continue to test. This means that what looks like a 6 to 8^Δ deviation when you start, may look more like an 18 to 20^Δ deviation by the time you're done. This brings us to the alternating prism cover test.

Alternating Prism Cover Test

The alternating prism cover test is the gold standard for measuring someone's maximum deviation. You typically do it right after you finish doing the cover-uncover test as described above. The idea is that you always have the occluder in front of one eye or the other, and, therefore, make it impossible for your patient to use the 2 eyes together. In this way, any –phoria that the patient may have will build to the maximum and add to whatever underlying –tropia he may have.

The alternating prism cover test starts out just like the cover-uncover test, and many clinicians just basically segue into it from the cover-uncover test. The patient should be looking at a distant target, such as a letter on the eye chart. Then cover one eye with an occluder like before. When you uncover that eye, instead of just taking the occluder away, as you did for the cover-uncover test, quickly use it to cover the other eye. Hold it there for a few seconds to let the patient pick up fixation with the newly uncovered eye, and then quickly move it back to the first eye again. As you keep repeating this process of covering first one eye and then the other, you may see the deviation start to build. Now it's time to measure it.

If you're holding the occluder in the right hand, you'll hold a prism with your left one to put in front of your patient's right eye. During this test, it doesn't matter which eye you put the prism in front of; do whatever is comfortable for you and your patient. If you see a deviation, place a prism in front of the eye so that the apex points toward the deviation. Continue to switch the occluder from eye to eye, being sure to give him 3 to 4 seconds to pick up fixation in between. If you still see a deviation even though there is a prism there, put that prism down and grab a different one being sure to keep the occluder up in front of one eye the whole time. You don't want the patient to be able to use both eyes together while you are rooting around in the drawer for another prism. Eventually, you'll have the proper prism, and your patient will have no deviation as you move the occluder back and forth. This is your endpoint. Note that if the patient has a combined horizontal (eso- or exo-) and vertical (hyper- or hypo-) deviation, you will need to be holding two prisms at the same time to reach this endpoint.

Your patient may have a deviation that is incongruous, meaning that it is different in different directions of gaze. For example, the deviation may be quite small when looking to the left, but very large when looking to the right. This usually occurs secondary to a problem with specific muscles (the right lateral rectus in this example). If this is the case, the alternating prism cover test needs to be repeated in all 6 cardinal positions of gaze. Also, if there is any incongruous vertical deviation, you will need to perform this test with the patient in a left and right head tilt position.

Finally, you'll have to repeat the alternating prism cover test when the patient is focusing on a near target. When recording the deviation, don't forget to write the prime sign (') showing that this represents a near deviation.

Maddox Rod

The cover-uncover test and alternating prism cover test are both used for patients who have *sensory deviations*. This means that the eyes can move in all directions, but that the brain just doesn't do it right for some reason. Another way to say this is that the motilities are correct, but the alignment is not. These tests rely on the patient being able to move the eye properly when the occluder is removed and, therefore, do not work well with patients who have restrictive motility problems. These patients have *motor deviations*, and the Maddox rod must be used to measure them.

The Maddox rod is a way to measure someone's deviation without his having to move his eye at all. It is a purely subjective test and relies on the patient's being able to respond to your questions. For this reason, it is not a good test for small children or patients with significant developmental delay.

The Maddox rod doesn't look like a rod at all. It is a ribbed, red plastic disc that is placed in front of one of your patient's eyes. Some Maddox rods are built into occluders, and other, smaller models will fit into trial frames. Most phoropters also have a Maddox rod that you can flip into place. Because the patient cannot really see through the Maddox rod, it is always a nonfusional test. For this reason, you will not be able to pick up subtle phorias with the Maddox rod test—it is an all or nothing test like the alternating prism cover test.

To perform this test, place a Maddox rod in front of one of your patient's eyes, and position a small light source (like a muscle light) across the room, or at least a few feet in front of him. The eye without the Maddox rod will see the small white light, and the eye with the Maddox rod will see a red line. If the ribs of the Maddox rod are arranged horizontally, the patient will see a vertical line; if the ribs are arranged vertically, he will see a horizontal line.

I always like to start with the ribs arranged horizontally so I can evaluate for an eso- or exo-deviation first.

With the ribs arranged horizontally in front of one eye, ask the patient if he or she can see a white light and a red, vertical line. If both eyes are working, both should be seen. Then merely ask him or her where the white light falls in relation to the red line. If the white light falls to the side of the red line, hold prism up in front of the non-Maddox rod eye until the white light falls on it. Then record the amount and direction of prism that it took to get the white light to sit atop the red line. Then turn the Maddox rod so the ribs are vertical, and repeat the test to look for a hypo- or hyper- deviation.

Because the Maddox rod test is such a disorienting test, you can't really measure a near deviation with it. However, because we're using this technique for patients with motility problems related to specific muscles (motor deviations), we will often need to repeat this test in different fields of gaze. Usually we do this by having the patient move his head rather than us moving the light source. Then just remember that a right head turn corresponds to a left gaze, a chin down position corresponds to an up gaze, and so on.

8

Slit Lamp Biomicroscopy

The slit lamp biomicroscope is more amazing than it appears at first blush. First, it magnifies whatever it is you are looking at. That is pretty basic, and I think most people understand how that works pretty well. Second, it illuminates whatever it is you're looking at. Again, this is pretty basic, although the skill of how much illumination to use and where to place it requires a significant amount of training. Third of all, it's *self-focusing*. That fact is very important; it means that *you* never have to actually focus your slit lamp. Whatever you're looking at is automatically brought into focus just by moving the oculars back and forth. This frees you up to concentrate on magnification and slit beam shapes and illumination without spending time with worrying about the focusing apparatus. That's pretty amazing considering that Gullstrand invented the modern slit lamp almost one hundred years ago.

So why a slit? Why not just have a regular light source hooked up to those oculars? What do we gain by having the light come out in a slit configuration? Well, as it turns out, a lot. As you will see below, the slit beam can be manipulated in a number of ways to maximize your view of what you're looking at. The hard part about examining the anterior segment of the eye relies on the fact that most of the things that you're called upon to examine are transparent. The conjunctiva, tear film, cornea, anterior chamber, pupil, lens, and anterior vitreous are all basically transparent. Add this to the fact that they're each very small, and you'll begin to see why we have to actually use a lot of "tricks" to be able to examine everything properly. Fortunately, through the magnification offered by the oculars in combination with the special illumination afforded by the slit beam, the slit lamp biomicroscope enables us to perform these tricks quite well—*as long as we know how to use it properly.*

MANIPULATING THE SLIT

The *height, width,* and *brightness* of the slit can each be altered by separate controls. If you think about it, all you really need to know how to change are those 3 specific qualities of the slit. Although different models of slit lamps may have the controls located in different places, they should all have some type of knob or dial to allow you to independently alter the height, width and brightness of the slit beam. You must familiarize yourself with the controls that will allow you to change these features. Go to a nearby slit lamp and turn it on. Hold up your finger or a piece of paper in the beam of the slit beam so that you can see the projected slit in focus through the oculars.

Find the control that allows you to manipulate the *height* of the slit. Turn it one way, and you'll notice that the slit gets tall. Turn it the other way, and the slit becomes short. Some slit lamps will have a measuring device somewhere that will tell you in fractions of a millimeter how high your slit beam is. Locate this scale, and observe how it records the height of the slit as you change it from short to tall.

Next, find the control that allows you to manipulate the *width* of the slit. Turn it one way, and the slit becomes very narrow (and eventually disappears). Turn it the other way, and the slit becomes fat until it eventually becomes a circle.

Finally, we can control the *brightness* of the slit. We can do that by placing various filters between the light source and the patient. When controls are set so that the slit is at its brightest, no filter is placed between the light source and the patient. If you position yourself on the receiving end of the slit (the patient's side), you will notice that in addition to being very bright, the slit actually emits warmth. When the slit is this bright, it is uncomfortable for the patient to keep his eye open unless the slit beam is made very narrow, thus, limiting the total energy reaching the patient. You can experiment with the various filters to see how they will make the slit appear dimmer or brighter. As a general rule, transparent structures (like the cornea and lens) should be viewed with bright light, while opaque structures (like the sclera and lids) should be viewed with dimmer light. Many clinicians will just leave the slit beam at an intermediate setting, but, in my opinion, this just combines the disadvantages inherent in both settings without actually maximizing on any of the advantages, therefore, I don't recommend it. Another good general rule to go by is that whenever you are using a lens to focus a slit beam on the retina, use a dim light.

There are other aspects of the slit beam that you can manipulate. One specific feature that is easily manipulated is the *color* of the slit. With one setting, you can make the slit green. This green filter is called a "red-free" filter and is useful in evaluating small hemorrhages in the retina, and the retinal nerve-fiber layer. It is also helpful in evaluating rose bengal staining of the cornea and conjunctiva. You can change the settings to make the slit cobalt blue (Wood's lamp). This feature is essential in evaluating fluorescein staining when looking at corneal or conjunctival abrasions.

Another thing we can control is the direction of the slit. We can make the slit beam come from the left, the right, or even straight ahead. More importantly, though, is that we can control the direction of the slit beam *independently* of the direction of the oculars. This means that we can continue to look straight into a patient's eyes while we move the slit beam from side to side. Conversely, we can shine the slit beam straight into someone's eyes while looking at them from one side or the other. The fact that these 2 factors can be controlled independently, while still never needing a separate focusing control, allows you to observe the eye in a very sophisticated method with minimal effort.

Another thing you can control is the magnification. Most slit lamps have a low (10x) and high (16x) magnification, although many of the newer models will have attachments that will allow even higher. It is not uncommon for the beginning clinician to use the highest magnification obtainable to see everything, and he will often find himself pressing his glasses (or corneas) against the oculars to get an even closer look. As you become proficient, you will find that some things (eyelids, conjunctiva) are best seen with low magnification, while others (corneal lesions, iris neovascularization) are best seen with high. Of course, there is a lot of personal preference inherent here; find a system you like and stick with it.

The last thing to find on the slit lamp is the fixation light. This is a small, dim light that automatically turns on when the slit lamp is turned on. It can be placed in front of the eye that you are not examining, thus giving the patient a target to look at. By using this light, you can help direct the patient's eye to a certain position and help bring an interesting piece of pathology into better view. It can also be used to help a patient keep his eye still for you while you are examining it.

APPRECIATING DEPTH

Just about everything you look at with the slit lamp is a 3-D object. Even the cornea and retina, which are both pretty thin and flat, have 3-D characteristics that are important to recognize while performing an examination. Fortunately, and this is no accident, the slit lamp is the ideal instrument for appreciating the depth of these, and other structures. There are 3 specific tricks to using the slit lamp that will enable you to appreciate the depth of the objects at which you are looking.

The first cue to depth you can call on when using the slit lamp is *stereopsis*. Most of you reading this text have 2 seeing eyes. Because of the way your eyes are positioned in the front of your head, separated by 5 to 7 cm, the image seen by the left eye is slightly different than that seen by the right eye. These images usually are not so different that the brain can not process them into something coherent, but they are different enough that the brain must perform some higher order processing to get them to make sense. What the brain does is to process the images together into a 3-D map through a process called stereopsis.

Slit lamps have 2 oculars to look through, one for your right eye and one for your left. If the objects in your field of view have any depth to them

Figure 8-1. In (a) and (b) slit beams are shown where the light source for the slit is off to the left about 45 degrees. (a) The object is caught in the left-hand side of the slit, so it must be located anteriorly. (b) The object is caught in the right-hand side of the slit, so it must be located posteriorly.

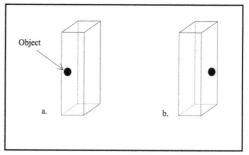

at all, the image seen by your right eye will be different than that seen by your left, and you will experience stereopsis and perceive the field in three dimensions. If you were to close one eye, the effect of stereopsis would disappear, and you would have to rely on other perceptual cues to appreciate the depth. Although stereopsis is a strong cue to the perception of depth, it is not the only one. Clinicians with only 1 eye, strabismus, amblyopia, or poor stereopsis for other reasons do quite well relying on the other cues.

The second trick we can perform to experience depth while using the slit lamp involves the direction of the incoming slit beam, and its relationship to the position of the oculars. Remember that a lot of the structures we look at through the slit lamp are basically transparent (eg, cornea, lens, vitreous). Sometimes we'll see an object that we know isn't supposed to be there, and we will say, "Now is that thing in the cornea, or the lens?" By changing the direction of the slit beam, we can usually answer that question pretty easily. We know the cornea sits anterior to the lens. Therefore, light from the slit beam will hit the cornea anterior to where it hits the lens. If we aim the slit beam straight into our patient's eye in the same direction that we are looking (coaxial), the slit on the cornea will overlap the slit on the lens, and very little detail can be seen. However, if we move the light source so that the slit comes from the left (and goes to the right), while keeping the oculars positioned so we're looking straight in, we see a different picture. Now we see 2 different segments of the slit beam, one in the cornea, and one in the lens. Of those 2 slits that you see, one is to the left, and the other to the right. We know from above that the beam of light is traveling from left to right, so the slit that's on the left (the corneal one) must be anterior to the slit that's on the right (the lens one).

That's a pretty obvious exercise to perform because everyone knows that the cornea is anterior to the lens. However, how do you figure out if the abnormality is anterior or posterior corneal stroma, or anterior or posterior lens? The same technique applies. Position the light source to the side so that the slit comes from left to right. If the abnormality is in the right-hand part of the slit beam, you know it has to be posterior, and if it's in the left-hand part, you know it's anterior (Figure 8-1).

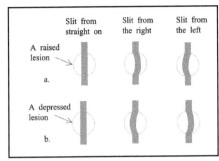

Figure 8-2. The position of the slit beam can be used to give cues to depth: (a) depicts a raised lesion and (b) depicts a depressed lesion. When the slit is aimed at the lesion from straight on, no cues to depth can be obtained from its shape. However, if the light source is moved from one side to the other, a lot of information about the nature of the lesion can be obtained.

The third and final trick involves the shape of the slit beam itself. The slit beam is shaped like a slit, and if it is projected onto a flat surface, it will still look like a slit. If it is projected onto an irregular surface, though, what happens? Well, that depends upon two specific things—the degree of irregularity of the surface, and the angle at which you're viewing it (Figure 8-2). Let's take an example where the slit beam is focused onto something that is bulging forward, like a tumor. If we shine the slit right straight onto it *in the same direction at which we're looking at it*, we probably will not be able to make out any 3-D characteristics. However, if we keep the oculars still, but move the light source so the slit comes in from the side, we perceive the slit as having a bump in it corresponding to the tumor. This effect, which is easily seen with a slit of light, does not work nearly as well when the light is in any non-slit configuration (such as a circle or square).

Similarly, we could aim the slit at something that represents a depression, such as an area of corneal thinning. If the light source and oculars were both aimed at the cornea from straight ahead, the slit would probably just look like a rectangular slit and not give you any cues as to the depression. Only when the light is moved to one side or the other, *while the oculars are kept still*, can the area of thinning be appreciated by the change in the shape of the slit. Thus, the shape of the slit alone, when positioned properly in relation to the location of the oculars, can give a lot of information as to the 3-D characteristics of the tissue being examined.

Thus, you have three basic cues for appreciating depth while using the slit lamp. The first involves the higher-order brain process called stereopsis, and depends upon the clinician possessing 2 functioning eyes, and using them to look through the two oculars of the slit lamp. The second involves the direction of the incoming light source, and is dependent upon the fact that the light beam can be moved so it comes in from one side or the other. The third involves the shape of the slit and is dependent upon the fact that the light source can be moved separately from the oculars. Now let's look at specific slit lamp techniques you can use to maximize your examination skills.

Figure 8-3. With direct illumination, the light source is positioned off to one side, and a bright slit beam is shone directly onto the object to be studied. The light is scattered in all directions by the object, and some of this scattered light finds its way back to the oculars, where it can be observed by the clinician.

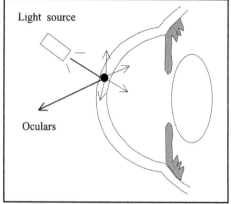

Specific Slit Lamp Techniques

There's more to using the slit lamp than shining a slit of light onto your patient's eye and looking at it with magnification through the oculars. Specific techniques, namely direct illumination, diffuse illumination, sclerotic scatter, retro-illumination, and specular microscopy, exist for viewing all of the different types of structures found within the eye. Each of these techniques has certain advantages over the others when used in specific situations. However, they each have certain inherent limitations, and it is just as important to understand the limitations for each technique, as it is the advantages. It is important to learn when to use which techniques to maximize the information you can get from your exam.

Direct Illumination

Direct illumination is the most tempting way to examine something when using the slit lamp. Many new clinicians who don't yet know how to properly use a slit lamp will use this technique almost exclusively, and, by doing so, will severely limit the amount of information they can obtain. Direct illumination does have its place in the anterior segment examination. It's just that it must be used in concert with all the other tricks at your disposal to be used properly.

Direct illumination is performed by placing a bright slit of light directly on whatever it is that you're trying to look at (Figure 8-3). It's effect is maximized when a bright, tall, thin slit is used and the oculars are set at maximal magnification. The light source should be positioned so that it is coming from the side, and the oculars should be positioned so that your view is straight-on.

The best use of direct illumination is to evaluate the *depth* of pathology within a transparent ocular structure. If a properly thin, bright beam is placed on the cornea, the true depth of a corneal abnormality can be determined. This works equally well to determine the location of lesions in the anterior chamber (cell and flare), lens (posterior subcapsular cataract) and anterior vitreous (cells, tobacco dust). It also works well to quantitate the amount of corneal thinning in inflammatory corneal diseases that result in focal loss of corneal thickness.

There are 2 specific limitations behind the technique of direct illumination. First, the light source aims the slit into the eye, in a direction similar to the direction of the observer's view. The observer, therefore, can only see light that is reflected back from the observed structures into the oculars of the slit lamp. If you are looking at a fairly transparent structure, most incoming light will pass through it with only a small amount of the light actually being reflected back to the oculars of the slit lamp. This system is inefficient in that many subtle abnormalities will be missed because they just do not reflect enough light back to the oculars.

The second limitation depends upon the brightness of the incoming slit beam. In order for direct illumination to be performed properly, a thin, *bright*, tall slit beam is placed on the structure you desire to see. Often, the beam is so bright, that when it is placed right on what you're trying to see, it will actually drown it out. When this occurs, the desired structure may actually be quite difficult to see. Sometimes this can be alleviated by dimming the slit, but often you will have to rely on the other techniques for better visualization.

Diffuse Illumination

Diffuse illumination is a second technique that many new clinicians may perform to the exclusion of the others. Diffuse illumination is performed by placing a dim, wide, and tall slit on an object and viewing it under low magnification. The light source is usually positioned so that the slit comes in from the side, while the oculars are positioned so the view is perpendicular to the iris plane. Diffuse illumination is best used for viewing opaque structures like the lids, conjunctiva, sclera, and iris.

The major advantage of diffuse illumination is in viewing surfaces of opaque objects. It is important to use a fairly dim slit so as not to drown what you are looking at with bright light, as can happen with direct illumination. By manipulating the angle of incidence of the incoming slit beam and narrowing the slit, topographic abnormalities of the surface such as pingueculae or nodules can be evaluated.

The major drawback to diffuse illumination is that it is not a good technique to use in evaluating transparent structures. It turns out that this isn't much of a drawback, though, because you have all the other techniques at your disposal for that.

Sclerotic Scatter

Sclerotic scatter is a technique that is not intuitively obvious. It depends upon total internal reflection, the same principle upon which fiberoptics is

Figure 8-4. With sclerotic scatter, a *bright*, wide slit is shone directly at the limbus. Most of the light is trapped within the cornea through total internal reflection, and, therefore, the cornea appears dark. However, when the light hits the opposite limbus or anything abnormal located within the corneal substance, it will scatter. Because some of the scattered light is directed back to the oculars, the abnormality is visible to the clinician.

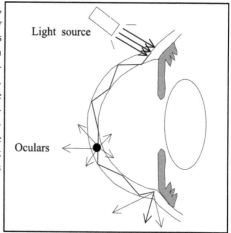

based. For more background on total internal reflection, refer to Chapter 9. At this time, all you need to know is that if light is shone into the cornea a certain way, it gets trapped within the corneal substance until it hits something which causes it to bounce out. That "something" can be the opposite limbus or, more importantly, it can be bits of pathology buried within the substance of the cornea.

To perform sclerotic scatter, shine a bright, fat, and tall slit right at the limbus at either the 3- or 9-o'clock position, and look at the entire cornea through low illumination (Figure 8-4). The idea is to trap as much light as you can within the substance of the cornea. If any of this light strikes anything abnormal, some of it will bounce back toward the oculars and you'll be able to see it.

The first thing you will notice when you set up correctly for sclerotic scatter is that the limbus lights up for 360 degrees. The second thing you will notice is that the normal cornea will appear pretty dark. This is because there really is not anything in the normal cornea that will cause the light to scatter and end up getting into your oculars and, therefore, it is optically quiet. However, if any pathology exists within the cornea, it will light up and be easy to locate. The third thing you'll notice is the patient may want to close his eye and pull back his head. You should be sensitive to the fact that sclerotic scatter depends on shining a lot of bright light into your patient's eye, and he may find it uncomfortable.

The major advantage of sclerotic scatter is that it is very sensitive for picking up pathology. The normal cornea is optically very quiet when using this technique. Even very subtle pathology, on the other hand, will light up when performing this technique, and will be surprisingly easy to see.

There are a few limitations to this procedure. The first is that it relies on very bright light, and patients with pathology that leaves them photophobic often find it very difficult to tolerate. The second limitation is that, although it is ideal for spotting pathology within the cornea, it does not tell you at which layer of the cornea the abnormality is located. That's fine, though, because once pathology is seen, it is easy enough to modify the slit beam and change over to direct illumination to further identify the problem. The third limitation is that it's only useful for corneal pathology, and can't be used to look at the lens, lids or other structures of the anterior segment.

Retro-Illumination

To perform retro-illumination, bounce the slit beam off something opaque (fundus or iris) behind what you're looking at which is transparent (cornea or lens). It is a powerful technique because it does away with one of the major shortcomings of the slit lamp—that the incoming light can never be much more than 90 degrees away from your view in. This is an important concept and deserves further explanation.

Think of how the microscope works. If you remember this device from high school science class, you'll remember that the ocular is located at the top, the light source is located at the bottom, and the specimen is located in-between. That's a great arrangement, because all the light from the bulb passes through the specimen, through the oculars, and into the observer's eye. This type of apparatus takes full advantage of the concept of *transmission*, the fact that the light that reaches the oculars has *transmitted through* whatever it is you're looking at.

Now think how different that is from the set up of the slit lamp. In the slit lamp, the light source and oculars are located on the same side. The specimen isn't located between them, so the oculars cannot collect transmitted light. Rather, the light is bounced off the specimen, and the oculars can only collect *reflected* or *scattered* light. Over 90% of the light generated by the lamp actually gets transmitted right through the ocular structures and is never seen by the observer. It's a pretty inefficient system, really.

Retro-illumination does away with this inefficiency and allows the observer to examine structures via transmitted light. It accomplishes this by shining light in through the pupil and allowing it to bounce off the fundus and return to the observer back out through the pupil (Figure 8-5). A short, wide, bright beam is aimed straight in through the pupil, perpendicular to the iris plane. The oculars are also set up so the view in is perpendicular to the iris plane. The incoming light passes through the cornea, anterior chamber, pupil, lens, and vitreous and bounces off the opaque fundus. A very large percentage of this light bounces right back through the vitreous, lens, pupil, anterior chamber, and cornea and ends up reaching the oculars of the slit lamp for your evaluation. The light that reaches your oculars has now passed right through all the transparent structures of the anterior segment on its way out. In this way, you can view structures via transmitted light rather than scattered or

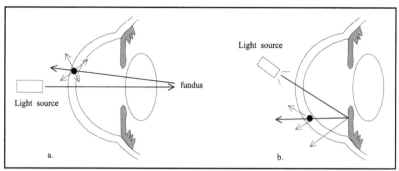

Figure 8-5. Retro-illumination is a technique that allows the observer to view a clear structure with light that has been transmitted through, rather than just bounced off it. In (a) the light from the slit lamp is shone through the pupil, reflected off the fundus, and transmitted through the lens and cornea. In (b) the light is reflected off the iris and transmitted through the cornea.

reflected light. In so doing, the sensitivity of the system goes up immensely, and even very subtle abnormalities can easily be seen.

The above technique describes shining light through the pupil and bouncing light off the fundus. The iris can be used to bounce light off in a similar way. When performing this technique, it is best to use a thinner, taller slit, and have it come in at a bit of an angle. What you will see when you have set it up right is a bright slit going in through the cornea, an area of lit-up iris behind it, and a second, more diffuse slit coming back through the cornea. Where you want to look is right between the 2 corneal slits in front of where the iris is lit up. Where the slit is passing through the cornea, direct illumination is going on, and we've already discussed how that can actually drown out important details. By focusing and looking between the 2 slits, you will maximize the sensitivity in examining subtle forms of corneal pathology.

Retro-illumination is an important way of spotting subtle pathology within the cornea, anterior chamber, lens, or vitreous. By manipulating the light source in such a way that you capture light that has passed through the pathology, rather than just bouncing off it, you maximize the chances of picking up things during your anterior segment examination. Limitations, of course, exist. The first limitation is that, as in sclerotic scatter, it depends upon a fairly bright slit beam, and photophobic patients may not tolerate it. When this is the case, you should try it again with a dimmer or smaller beam.

The second limitation is that the depth of the lesion cannot be evaluated. The light is bounced of the fundus (which is in the back of the eye) and is collected in the oculars (which sit a few centimeters in front). Pathology that lies anywhere between these 2 structures will show up using this technique, and you usually will not be able to tell whether the abnormality seen is in the vitreous, lens, anterior chamber, cornea, or tear film.

Specular Microscopy

The last slit lamp technique, specular microscopy, warrants a quick review of some optical principles. As you no doubt remember from reading Chapter 3, when light passes from a medium of one refractive index to a medium of another, it may be bent, or refracted. However, that is not all that goes on at the interface. Not only is some of the light refracted, but some of it is absorbed, and some is reflected. The eye is efficient at what it does, so very little incoming visible light is normally absorbed or reflected, while the overwhelming majority of it gets refracted as it passes through the cornea and lens on its way toward the retina. We can, however, take advantage of the small amount that is reflected by using the slit lamp technique known as specular microscopy.

For specular microscopy, a bright, tall, moderately thin slit beam is projected from about 45 degrees off to one side. The oculars are positioned so the view in is perpendicular to the iris plane, and high magnification is used. When looking at the endothelium of the cornea, the slit is aimed at the posterior corneal surface and is bounced off the refractive interface between the cornea and the aqueous humor. If the interface is perfectly smooth, no detail will be seen at the interface with slit lamp magnification (with a special instrument called a specular microscope, higher magnification together with this technique will allow for study of the morphology of individual epithelial cells). However, if pathology such as Descemet's folds or guttatae exists, it will easily appear as bright and dark irregularities in the reflected surface.

A similar technique can be used when looking at the anterior surface of the cornea. Again, a bright, moderately wide slit beam is used, and the light source is set up so the slit comes from off to one side. This time, the refractive interface is at the junction of the tear film and air. When the slit is positioned properly, the surface anatomy can be evaluated. Abnormalities such as epithelial defects, anterior scars, and band keratopathy can easily be seen through this technique. Although specular microscopy is best used for evaluating features of the cornea, it can also be used for examining different aspects of the lens.

THE ANTERIOR SEGMENT EXAMINATION

Now let's put together all these slit lamp techniques to perform an anterior segment examination. We start at the front, and work our way posteriorly.

Eyelids and Eyelashes

As we examine from front to back, the first thing we come upon are the eyelids and eyelashes. Often overlooked, these are important because they are often responsible for complaints associated with redness, irritation, itchiness, and so on. They are best viewed using diffuse illumination under low magnification.

When handling the lids, you should get in the habit of using a cotton-tipped applicator (CTA) rather than your fingers. This may keep you from picking up an infectious organism from one patient, and spreading it to all the patients you see later on that day. If the patient has a red eye, or other pathology that may seem contagious, be sure to throw the CTA away after examining the infected eye. This means that if you examine the right eye first, and this is the red one, throw the CTA away and grab a clean one before you examine the left eye. This simple act should keep you from turning a monocular infection into a bilateral one.

To examine a lower lid, gently apply the CTA 4 to 5 mm below the lid margin and ask the patient to look up. By doing this, you will automatically expose the lid margin, with its full complement of meibomian gland orifices and eyelash follicles, for you to examine. When you're done looking at the lower lid, place the CTA gently against the upper lid about 5 or 6 mm above the lid margin and ask the patient to look down. This maneuver will bring the meibomian glands and lash follicles of the upper lid into view. In this way, you can easily examine the patient to look for blepharitis, rosacea, growths, tumors, and other sources of eyelid pathology. The back side of the lids is covered with conjunctiva, so we will discuss that in the next section.

Conjunctiva and Sclera

The next things to look at are the conjunctiva and sclera. The *palpebral* conjunctiva lines the back surfaces of all 4 eyelids, the *bulbar* conjunctiva covers the sclera of the anterior part of the eyeball, and the *forniceal* conjunctiva lies in between (in the fornix). You should examine a patient's entire conjunctiva with diffuse illumination, using a tall, wide, dim beam under low magnification. Start with the bulbar conjunctiva. Ask your patient to look temporally to examine his nasal bulbar conjunctiva, look nasally to examine his temporal bulbar conjunctiva, look up (while holding down his lower lid with a CTA) to examine his inferior bulbar and forniceal conjunctiva, and look down (while holding up his lower lid with a CTA) to examine his superior bulbar conjunctiva.

The palpebral conjunctiva of the lower lid can be seen by holding the lid with a CTA and asking the patient to look upwards. The tarsus is so small in the lower lids (about 4 mm high), that its conjunctival surface can usually be seen just by doing as I just described. This, unfortunately, is not the case for the upper eyelids, where the tarsus is a full 10 to 11 mm high. To see the conjunctival surface of the upper eyelids, the lid has to be "flipped." To flip a lid, place a CTA (the wooden end actually works better here because it's smaller than the cotton tipped end) so that it is oriented parallel to both the floor and the iris plane, and located about 10 mm above the lid fissure. By placing it here, you have laid the CTA so it is up against the top surface of your patient's tarsal plate at the level of the lid crease. Then ask the patient to look down while you get a hold of some eyelashes with your free hand.

Pull the lashes up while you press the CTA slightly down and against the globe (not too hard here). If the CTA is located in the right place, the tarsus will flip right over it and you'll be looking at a 10 mm expanse of upper palpebral conjunctiva. The patient will be most comfortable during this procedure if he is reminded to look down the whole time. The lid will usually flip back on its own when you let go of the lashes, but sometimes you have to coax it back to the proper position with your fingertip.

The sclera lies underneath the bulbar conjunctiva. There usually aren't a lot of details of the sclera that are easily seen through the conjunctiva. Be aware of areas of thinning or nodularity. Also be aware that some cases of a red eye are secondary to scleritis, so you will have to recognize inflammation of the sclera and be able to differentiate it from inflammation of the conjunctiva (conjunctivitis) and inflammation of the episclera (episcleritis). Because the sclera is an opaque structure, it, too, is best seen under diffuse illumination using a tall, wide, dim slit under low magnification.

Tear Film

Do not forget about the tear film. Many patients have complaints of eye pain and irritation closely related to tear film dysfunction. It is important to evaluate the volume of the tear film as well as the presence or absence of any debris that may be floating in it.

The best way to see the tear film is with specular reflection. Place a high, medium width, and bright slit right on the tear film and move the light source so the beam is coming from about 45 degrees off to one side. Try to judge the tear film volume by looking at the meniscus the tears make with the lower lid margin. A patient with aqueous tear film deficiency will likely have a low meniscus, while a patient with epiphora will have a high one.

Next, you need to evaluate the clarity of the tear film. The normal tear film is fairly optically empty which means there are not a lot of details to make out in it. Actually, it is so optically empty and so thin that it is often difficult to see at all. Many abnormalities of the tear film, however, make the tear film visible. The best example of this phenomenon can be seen in patients with Meibomian gland dysfunction. These patients will often have a film of oily debris or soaps (which are breakdown products of the oils) floating on the surface of their tear film, thus making it quite visible. Other patients may have bits of eyeliner, eyelashes, or other items floating in their tears.

Because the tear film is so thin and optically empty, sometimes it may be difficult to tell whether an abnormality is in the tear film or on the corneal surface. When this is the case, merely ask your patient to blink. If the abnormality is truly corneal, it should stay put. However, if it lies in the tear film, it will move around in the tears with the motion of the lids.

While you are examining the tear film, you can evaluate its quality by measuring the tear film break-up time (BUT). Patients with some dry eye type disorders may make enough tears, but will develop dry spots on the surface of their eyes between blinks. This is usually due to the problems with the quality of the tear film, and is related to the interactions between its water, mucin, and oil layers. To measure a tear film BUT, place some fluorescein in the tear film, use the cobalt blue filter, focus the slit beam on a patient's tear film using sclerotic scatter, ask him to blink, and then stare with his eyes open. Then, count to yourself and watch for the development of dry patches, which will look like black patches in the green field of fluorescein. In a normal eye, there should still be no dry patches at 10 seconds. If a patient develops dry patches earlier than this, just record how long it took for them to develop. For instance, if it took 6 seconds for dry spots to develop, record, "tear film BUT=6 seconds."

Cornea

A lot of corneal disease is pretty subtle, so you want to start your exam with the techniques that are most sensitive to subtle pathology. The first of these is sclerotic scatter. To perform this, place a bright, wide, high beam at the limbus, and see if any abnormalities light up within the corneal substance. A second technique you can perform for the same effect is retro-illumination. Either of these techniques should give you a good idea of the general location of any abnormalities residing within the cornea. As discussed before, however, neither of these techniques will let you know the corneal depth of a lesion.

Next, examine the corneal surface using specular reflection. Place a high, moderately wide, bright slit on the cornea, and move the oculars so that the corneal epithelium is in focus. Move the light source so that it is coming from one side about 45 degrees or so, and use high magnification. If you feel you are missing a lot of the surface detail, either dim the slit a little, or work on fine tuning the focus. Through this technique, you should be able to make out any abnormalities in the ocular surface.

If you are worried about an epithelial defect, you may want to touch a fluorescein strip to the inferior tear film, ask the patient to blink, and view it with the cobalt blue light. Any areas of the cornea that now glow green may correspond to an area of epithelial defect. Be careful of mucus that will stain green with fluorescein and may make you think you are looking at a big epithelial defect. If you suspect that you are looking at mucus, just ask the patient to blink, and the mucus blob should move with the blink (an epithelial defect won't). Also, when you stain the cornea with fluorescein for diagnostic reasons, use the paper strips; don't use the liquid fluorescein bottles that you use to measure the intraocular pressure. The total amount of fluorescein in each drop is too high to perform a subtle slit lamp examination.

You next want to evaluate the corneal stroma. At this point, you should have some idea of where in the cornea any pathology lies, because you've already located it with sclerotic scatter and retro-illumination. All that's left to do is to figure out the level of the cornea that's involved. The best way to do this is through direct illumination. Shine a bright, tall, paper-thin slit on the cornea so it's coming from the side, and set the oculars so you're looking through high magnification. By putting the slit right on those areas where you saw abnormalities through sclerotic scatter and retro-illumination, you should be able to evaluate their depth in the corneal stroma. Remember, if the slit is shone in from left to right, the more posterior corneal findings will be found in the right-hand part of the slit, while the more anterior ones will be found in the left-hand part. If this doesn't make sense to you, reread the section on direct illumination.

After finding the depths of all those stromal abnormalities, it's time to evaluate the posterior corneal surface, which is made up of Descemet's membrane and the endothelium. The best way to evaluate this layer is through specular reflection. Broaden the slit a little from how you had it for direct illumination, but otherwise keep everything the same. Next, push the focus of the oculars forward a little so you're focused right at the interface between the endothelium and the aqueous humor. If you've set it up right, you should be able to see any abnormalities in the posterior corneal surface quite easily.

Anterior Chamber

The next structure to look at as we move our way posteriorly, is the anterior chamber. The anterior chamber is a space bordered anteriorly and laterally by the cornea, and posteriorly by the iris and pupil. It is normally filled with aqueous humor. A healthy aqueous humor is optically empty, which means that light goes right through it without any of it being reflected back for you to see anything with a slit lamp. Therefore, anything that can be seen within the anterior chamber must, by definition, be abnormal.

The best way to visualize things in the anterior chamber using the slit lamp is by an adaptation of direct illumination. Make the slit a small 1 mm x 1 mm, bright square, and shine it in from about 45 degrees to one side. Be sure to set the light very bright, to look through with high magnification, and to set up the focus so you're looking in the anterior chamber. If you're focused on the cornea, you need to push it back a little bit, and if you're focused on the iris, you need to pull it forward. Any visible abnormalities in the anterior chamber will show up directly in the path of the slit.

Sometimes you'll see *cells* floating. If the patient has a hyphema, these cells will be red blood cells, and will actually look red in the white slit beam. If the patient has inflammation (iritis, keratitis), the cells will be white blood cells and will appear white. In either case, you will only be able to see the cells located directly in the slit beam, and only if you're properly focused to look in the anterior chamber. Most of the time, these cells will be floating in the slit beam much like dust particles will float in a shaft of sunlight. The amount of cells is graded on a 1-to-4 plus system. One way to do this is as follows. If there are 10 to 20 cells in a 1 mm x 1 mm slit beam, it's 1+ cell; if there are 20 to 30 cells, it's 2+ cell; if there are greater than 30 cells, it's 3+ cell; and if there is a layered hypopyon or hyphema, it's 4+ cell.

Sometimes, the aqueous humor will appear slightly hazy. The normal aqueous, remember, is essentially optically empty which means that you cannot even see the slit beam as it traverses the anterior chamber. If you can make out the slit beam at all, the patient has some degree of *flare*. The visual effect of flare is seen because of protein that has leaked into the anterior chamber from anterior segment inflammation. The slit beam is scattered enough by the floating protein particles that it becomes visible when seen through the magnification of the oculars. Flare is graded on a 1– to 4+ system, as is cell, its anterior chamber partner. One+ flare means that you can barely make out the slit beam. Four+ flare means that there is solidified fibrin within the anterior chamber. Two+ and 3+ flare lie somewhere in between.

When evaluating a patient for flare, you must be aware of one confounding thing. Any patient who has had fluorescein applied to his tear film (and that includes anyone who's had his pressure taken via applanation tonometry, remember) will appear to have flare. Fluorescein penetrates the cornea easily to enter the anterior chamber. Once it's there, it is not as optically quiet as normal aqueous humor, and will allow the slit beam to be seen, thus imitating flare. Therefore, if you are at all concerned about your patient having flare, it's imperative that you examine the anterior chamber before administrating any fluorescein to the tear film.

Iris

The next structure to evaluate is the iris. The iris is opaque, so the best way to see abnormalities in it is through diffuse illumination. Place a wide, tall, dim (although bright works well here, too) beam on the iris, and view it through either low or high illumination. Look for changes in pigmentation and texture. If you feel the patient has a mass involving the iris, have the slit beam come from the side to better appreciate the depth of the lesion (see Figure 8-2).

It is also important to document abnormalities in the iris that are known as iris trans-illumination defects (TIDs). The normal iris is completely opaque. No light passes through it except at the pupil. Some conditions, such as albinism and pigment dispersion syndrome, will allow light to pass through the iris stroma. Surgical procedures, especially peripheral iridotomies, may also cause a hole that will allow light to pass right through the iris. The best way to visualize TIDs is through retro-illumination—preferably while the patient is still undilated. Take a short, wide, bright slit, and aim it straight through the pupil. If there are any iris TIDs, you will see them as areas of red reflex showing through the iris stroma. Be sure to focus on the iris while you are performing this technique. Remember that if you are looking for old peripheral iridotomies, they are usually placed far superiorly, and you will probably have to lift the lid to see them.

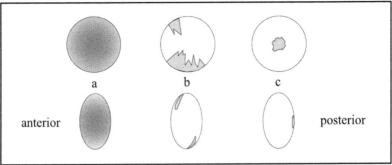

Figure 8-6. Different types of cataracts as viewed from the front (top row) and the side (bottom row). (a) Nuclear sclerosis. (b) Cortical spoking. (c) Posterior subcapsular.

Lens

When viewed with the slit lamp, the layers of the lens are easily seen. Because of all the layers, the crystalline lens resembles an onion. Any abnormalities in the lens are called cataract, although many clinicians reserve this term for abnormalities that cause visual complaints (usually either glare or decreased acuity). Cataract takes on one or a combination of three specific forms: nuclear sclerosis, cortical spoking, or posterior sub-capsular (Figure 8-6). *Nuclear sclerosis* (NS) is seen as a yellowing or darkening of the central part of the lens. Patients can often tolerate this for years without becoming overtly symptomatic—similar to wearing sunglasses all the time. *Cortical spoking* (C/S) is seen as white opacities within the lens cortex—usually located peripherally in a spoke-like configuration. Because these normally start peripherally, they also may be present for years before they become symptomatic. *Posterior subcapsular* (PSC) changes are normally seen at the posterior pole of the lens—right in the center of the pupil. Due to their location, even fairly small posterior subcapsular opacities may be quite bothersome to the patient. Posterior subcapsular cataract is the type that develops in diabetics and patients taking corticosteroids.

The lens can be evaluated through a combination of retro-illumination and direct illumination. It is imperative that the pupil be dilated to properly perform an examination of the crystalline lens. Nuclear sclerosis does not usually have any specific findings other than an overall color change to the central part of the lens. Because of this, it is the most difficult type of lens change for the beginning clinician to appreciate through slit lamp examination. You may have to look at a fair number of normal lenses before you can appreciate a nuclear sclerotic lens.

Cortical spoking and posterior subcapsular cataract show up quite well with retroillumination. Make the slit beam a very small, bright square, and shine it directly into the pupil. If you focus on the lens, any abnormalities in the red-reflex should correspond to cataractous lenticular changes. You may have to move the slit beam around a little bit to see the whole lens because the incoming bright slit of light will drown out areas of the red reflex, thus hiding important potential areas of pathology.

Once any abnormalities in the lens are seen through retro-illumination, try to figure out their depth through direct illumination. Place a tall, thin, bright slit on the cornea so that it is coming from the side, and look with high magnification. Find the bits of pathology that you saw with retro-illumination, and try to figure out whether they are anterior subcapsular, anterior cortical, nuclear (central), posterior cortical, or posterior subcapsular. Remember, if the slit beam is coming from the left side, anything seen in the left-hand part of the slit will be more anterior than anything seen in the right-hand part of the slit (see Figure 8-1).

Anterior Vitreous

The most posterior structure that you should be able to evaluate during the anterior segment examination is the anterior vitreous. Through a dilated pupil, with the slit lamp, you should be able to see the vitreous located immediately posterior to the crystalline lens. The best way to look at it is with direct illumination using a tall, bright, thin slit beam positioned so the light is coming from the side. The first thing you will notice is that the vitreous isn't as optically empty as the aqueous humor. It has a swirling consistency that is easily seen in the slit beam.

Most abnormalities of the anterior vitreous present as cells or debris during slit lamp examination. As in the anterior chamber, cells in the vitreous may be either red blood cells (vitreous hemorrhage) or white blood cells (vitritis or posterior uveitis). Again, it is documented on a scale from 1+ to 4+. Debris, is more diverse in nature, and can stem from a number of etiologies. Tobacco dust is a specific form of vitreous debris that represents pigment released into the vitreous during a retinal detachment or tear.

RECORDING YOUR FINDINGS

There are many ways to record your anterior segment examination findings. Many clinicians, especially those of us in private practice who do not see the sheer volume of pathology of those in academia, may just write out the results with a series of abbreviations. An example of this is, "SLE: l/l,a c/s, k, a/c, i, l, v nl OU," which is shorthand for, "slit lamp exam: lids/lashes/adnexa, cornea/sclera, cornea, anterior chamber, iris, lens, vitreous normal both eyes." It serves the dual purpose of getting the point across while not taking up a lot of space in the chart. This type of nomenclature is adequate for normal exams, but is inadequate for recording pathology.

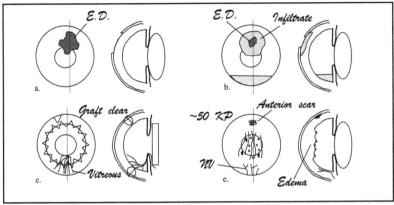

Figure 8-7. Four examples of slit lamp drawings are shown. (a) The area of epithelial defect is drawn in green. (b) The small area of epithelial defect is drawn in green while the larger anterior infiltrate is drawn in orange. The hypopyon is colored orange. (c) The stitches of the corneal transplant are drawn in black. The vitreous strands in the anterior chamber are shown in green. Note that this patient has a PCL that is also drawn in green. (d) This patient has HSV disciform endotheliitis. Where the cornea is thickened is colored blue, and the underlying keratic precipitates are drawn in orange. The anterior stromal scar, evidence of prior HSV infection, is colored black. Note that anterior and lateral views of each drawing must be made to fully describe the pathology. The smaller central circle in each picture corresponds to the pupil—note the PI in (c).

Table 8-1

WARING AND LAIBSON'S SYSTEM FOR DRAWING SLIT LAMP FINDINGS

Black	Scar, degeneration, suture, contact lens (dotted line)
Blue	Edema, Descemet's folds
Brown	Pigment, iris
Red	Blood, rose bengal
Green	Epithelial defects, lens, IOL, vitreous
Orange or yellow	Infiltrate, hypopyon, keratic precipitates.

The best way to record pathology is with detailed drawings (Figure 8-7). Waring and Laibson have written an excellent article on a systematic method for recording your anterior segment findings via drawings[1] (Table 8-1). There are a few specific keys to their system. First, always draw your findings from both the front and the side. What you are looking at, remember, is 3-D, and you just cannot do it any justice by merely drawing it from the front. By drawing your findings from the side as well as the front, you can easily record areas of corneal thinning or edema, IOL capture, vitreous in the anterior chamber, iris tumors, the depth of corneal infiltrates, and a myriad of other findings.

Second, be consistent with the colors. Your clinic may want you to do it a specific way, but Table 8-1 presents a general rule.

References

1. Waring GO, Laibson PR: A systematic method of drawing corneal pathologic conditions. *Arch Ophthalmol.* 1977;95:1540–1542.

9

Gonioscopy

THE ANTERIOR CHAMBER ANGLE

The anterior chamber angle is made up of all the structures formed at the junction of the cornea, sclera, and iris. It is located at the corneo-scleral limbus. From the front, the anterior chamber angle does not look too special—the sclera, covered by the episclera and conjunctiva, ends, and the cornea begins. All of the important structures lie beneath the surface.

If we could position ourselves so that we were standing on the iris and look toward the angle, we would see the anterior chamber angle (Figure 9-1). Starting anteriorly and moving posteriorly, the first structure we'd see would be the *cornea*. The cornea is, for the most part, transparent. It is dome-shaped with its apex in the center of the visual axis and base at the anterior chamber angle. From our iris-eyed view, the posterior cornea meets the sclera at a specific line. Microscopically, this line correlates with the furthest peripheral extent of Descemet's membrane. Grossly, it is a white line seen at the base of the clear cornea. This white line, when viewed gonioscopically, is called *Schwalbe's line*.

Schwalbe's line can always be located gonioscopically because it falls at the tip of the "corneal light wedge" (Figure 9-2). If you shine a bright, thin slit beam at the angle structures, you should see two corneal reflections, an anterior one and a posterior one. These 2 reflections make up the "corneal light wedge" and correspond to the anterior and posterior surfaces of the cornea. Because the cornea ends at Schwalbe's line, these 2 corneal light reflections will always meet there.

Immediately posterior to Schwalbe's line is a band, which is usually brown in color. This band, called the *trabecular meshwork*, is the porous tissue through which aqueous humor must pass on its way out of the eye. In some patients, the trabecular meshwork will have collected a lot of pigment, and will be easy to see. However, many patients will have minimal to no pigment, making the trabecular meshwork difficult to make out when viewed

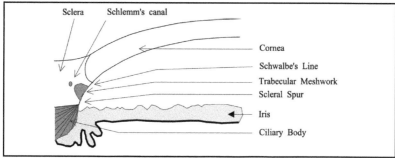

Figure 9-1. The anterior chamber angle is made up of the sclera, cornea, Schwalbe's line, trabecular meshwork, scleral spur, iris, and ciliary body. Note that Schwalbe's line corresponds to the posterior aspect of Descemet's membrane, and the scleral spur is the part of the sclera where the ciliary body inserts. The trabecular meshwork sits in a cavity between Schwalbe's line and the scleral spur.

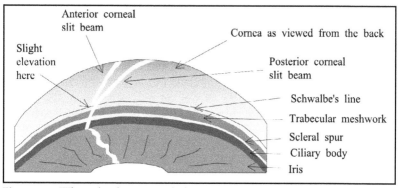

Figure 9-2. When a bright, narrow slit beam is projected through the cornea, 2 linear projections appear corresponding to the anterior and posterior corneal surfaces. These 2 beams of light make up the "corneal light wedge." They meet at Schwalbe's line.

gonioscopically. In these patients, Schwalbe's line should be found first, and the trabecular meshwork identified by the fact that it lies immediately posterior to Schwalbe's line.

The *scleral spur* is located posterior to the trabecular meshwork. Like Schwalbe's line, the scleral spur is a white line that can be identified when viewed gonioscopically. The scleral spur is an important anatomic landmark because it serves as the insertion of the ciliary body and iris root. Medications such as pilocarpine function to decrease intraocular pressure by causing contraction of the ciliary body. This increased ciliary body tone pulls on the scleral spur thus changing the shape of the trabecular meshwork resulting in decreased resistance to outflow of aqueous.

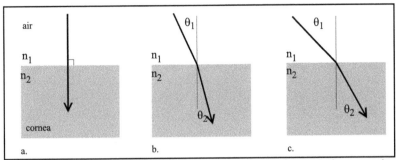

Figure 9-3. (a) When light passes from a medium of one refractive index to another perpendicularly to the interface, it is not bent. (b & c) When light passes unperpendicularly to the interface, it is bent in such a way that $(n_1)(\sin\theta_1) = (n_2)(\sin\theta_2)$. Note that because n_2 (which represents the refractive index of the cornea) is greater than n_1 (which represents the refractive index of air), θ_1 will always be greater than θ_2.

Inserting on the scleral spur is the next important anterior chamber angle structure, the *ciliary body*. The ciliary body is a fairly densely pigmented structure and therefore appears brown when viewed gonioscopically. It is located at the iris root, and is responsible for many functions including lens support, accommodation, and production of aqueous humor.

The one remaining angle structure that must be recognized is the *iris*. For the most part, like the cornea, the iris can be well visualized via slit lamp biomicroscopy. However, the peripheral aspects of the iris are better seen through gonioscopy. Gonioscopy will also allow for better observation of 3-D abnormalities of the iris such as tumors and cysts.

TOTAL INTERNAL REFLECTION

You may be asking yourself why you have to perform gonioscopy, and why not just look at the anterior chamber angle structures with the slit lamp. To answer this question, you have to remember back to Snell's Law. Snell's Law, remember, states that light will bend when traveling from a medium of one refractive index to a medium of another, *provided that the light crosses the interface in any direction other than perpendicular* (Figure 9-3). The equation can be written as $(n_1)(\sin\theta_1) = (n_2)(\sin\theta_2)$ where n_1 is the refractive index of the first medium, and n_2 is the refractive index of the second medium. As light passes from a medium with a low refractive index (such as air) to a medium with a higher refractive index (such as the tear film, cornea, or aqueous humor), the light is always bent toward the perpendicular. This means that the angle of the light on the air side is always going to be larger than the angle of the light on the corneal side. If you think about it, at some certain angle of light less than 90 degrees on the corneal side, the angle

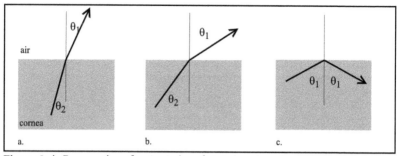

Figure 9-4. Because the refractive index of air is less than the refractive index of the cornea, angle θ_1 is always going to be greater than angle θ_2 (a & b). At some point (c), while θ_1 is still less than 90 degrees, θ_2 is going to be greater than 90 degrees. Total internal reflection occurs at this point, and light cannot escape the anterior chamber.

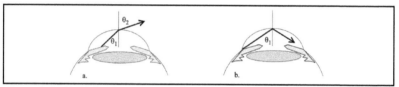

Figure 9-5. (a) Light that originates from the mid-iris intersects the cornea with a small enough angle (θ_1) that θ_2 is less than 90 degrees and that part of the iris can be visualized from outside the eye. (b) Light that originates from the anterior chamber angle structures intersects the cornea with such a large angle (θ_1) that total internal reflection occurs, and these structures cannot be visualized with simple slit lamp biomicroscopy.

of light on the air side has got to be greater than 90 degrees. At this point, light originating within the anterior chamber cannot escape; instead, it gets reflected back into the anterior chamber (Figure 9-4). This phenomenon is called *total internal reflection*.

The anterior chamber angle structures are located so far peripherally that light that comes from them hits the corneal endothelium at a very obtuse angle (Figure 9-5). The angle is so large that the light cannot overcome the difference in refractive index from the cornea (1.376) to the air (1.00), and thus gets reflected back into the anterior chamber. So, as long as there is air against the corneal tear film, the anterior chamber angle structures cannot be directly observed through the slit lamp. We perform gonioscopy to overcome this.

Different Methods of Gonioscopy

The principles behind all types of gonioscopy are similar. Basically, we want to eradicate total internal reflection so that the anterior chamber angle structures can be visualized. To do this, Snell's Law must somehow

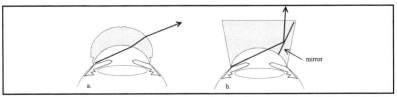

Figure 9-6. (a) The Koeppe lens is an example of a direct gonioscopic lens. It is little more than a molded piece of plastic that does away with total internal reflection by replacing the air-tear interface with an air-plastic one. (b) The Goldmann and Zeiss lenses are examples of indirect gonioscopic lenses. They, too, replace the air-tear interface with an air-plastic or air-glass one. However, the mirror allows light leaving the angle structures to exit the lens at an angle suitable for viewing through a slit lamp.

be manipulated and taken advantage of. Snell's Law, remember, states that $(n_1)(\sin\theta_1)=(n_2)(\sin\theta_2)$. Under physiologic conditions of the eyeball, n_1 equals the refractive error of the cornea-aqueous-tear film, and θ_1 equals the angle of light coming from the chamber angle structures. Neither of these 2 things can be simply altered in the eye clinic. The angle θ_2 is what we need to eventually change; we need to make this less than 90 degrees so that light can escape the anterior chamber and we may see it. All that's left to change, then, is n_2. This is a fairly easy thing to do. Normally, air is up against the tear film, and it is the difference in refractive errors between air and tears (n_1 and n_2) that allows total internal reflection to occur. When performing gonioscopy, material with a refractive index closer to that of the cornea is placed up against the tear film. This simple act allows light that hits the interface with a much greater angle to escape the anterior chamber. In this way, total internal reflection is overcome, and the anterior chamber angle structures can be visualized. Let's look at some examples of what we can place on the cornea to accomplish this.

Koeppe Lens

The Koeppe lens was one of the first gonioscopy lenses developed. It is a molded piece of plastic that can be placed on the cornea thus eliminating the air/cornea refractive interface (Figure 9-6a). There are no mirrors built into the Koeppe lens, and for this reason, Koeppe lens gonioscopy is referred to as *direct* gonioscopy.

To perform gonioscopy with a Koeppe lens, the patient must be lying down in a supine position. A solution, such as saline, artificial tears, or carboxymethylcellulose, is placed on the surface of the lens that is to be placed on the cornea. Anesthetic drops are placed on the surface of the eye, and the lens is positioned into place on the cornea and held in place by the lids. A fiberoptic illuminator can then be used to illuminate any part of the angle that you wish to observe. By walking around the patient and repositioning the light source, the entire 360 degrees of anterior chamber angle can be visualized.

Because Koeppe lens gonioscopy does not require the use of a slit lamp, it is often used on small children who may not sit at the slit lamp. The fact that this lens is not used in conjunction with a slit lamp is one of its major disadvantages. If magnification of the angle structures is desired, you must use a separate magnification system. Another disadvantage to the Koeppe lens is that the patient must be supine in order to perform it properly.

Goldmann Lens

The Goldmann lens was invented to overcome a lot of the limitations inherent in the Koeppe lens system. Like the Koeppe lens, the Goldmann lens places a piece of plastic (or glass) against the surface of the cornea to alleviate the gross difference in refractive error between the cornea and the air. However, unlike the Koeppe lens, the Goldmann lens has a mirror, which allows light that is projected perpendicularly to the iris plane to be bent into the anterior chamber angle (Figure 9-6b). This feature allows the Goldmann lens to be used in conjunction with a slit lamp with the patient sitting up.

Because the mirror is flat, and only reflects about 90 degrees of the angle on the opposite side, a few principles must be considered when using the Goldmann lens. First of all, everything seen in the mirror is the mirror image of what you are observing. That means that if you are looking into the mirror while it is positioned at the temporal aspect of a patient's eye, you are actually examining the angle structures located nasally. However, up is still up, and down is still down, unlike what happens with the indirect ophthalmoscope, as we'll learn in Chapter 11. The other thing to consider is that because the mirror only reflects around 90 degrees of angle, it must be rotated on the patient's eye in order to see the entire 360 degrees of angle.

When you properly use the Goldmann lens, the patient should be seated at the slit lamp. Place a numbing drop in his eye, and put a generous lubricating drop onto the corneal surface of the Goldmann lens. Next, tell the patient: "This special lens is going to sit between your lids and help me keep your eyes open— try not to blink it out— concentrate on looking at my ear with your other eye." Next, gently pull down the patient's lower lid and ask him to look up (which will raise the upper lid automatically). Place the bottom of the lens into his lower cul-de-sac, and place the upper part of the lens under his upper lid.

If you're using a one-mirror lens, find the mirror. If you're using a 3-mirror lens, find the gonioscopic mirror (the other 2 are for posterior segment examination) that is the one with the curved edge (the "thumbnail" shaped lens). I find it best to use high magnification and a bright, narrow slit beam. Be consistent and systematic when performing gonioscopy—always look at different quadrants in the same order. The best quadrant to start with is usually the inferior quadrant (the superior mirror, remember) because it will have the most pigment and will often be a little more open than the others, thus making the angle easier to examine. One of the systems I recommend is to look at quadrants in alphabetical order (inferior, nasal, superior, temporal); this way you'll never forget to look at any one area. When you are all done, remove the lens and repeat with the other eye.

Zeiss 4-Mirror Lens

The Zeiss 4-mirror lens, like the Goldmann lens, contains mirrors, and, therefore, is a form of indirect gonioscopy (Figure 9-6b). In almost every regard, the Zeiss lens functions exactly like the Goldmann lens. There are, however, a few distinct differences.

First of all, the part of the Zeiss lens that actually touches the cornea is smaller than that part of the Goldmann lens. What this means to you is that you will not have to manipulate the lids as much to get the lens in there. A second difference is that the Zeiss lens has 4 gonio-mirrors to the Goldmann lens' one. This means to you will be able to view all 360 degrees (90 degrees at a time, still) without rotating the lens. You just have to move the slit beam from one mirror to the other.

Otherwise, the use of the Zeiss lens is similar to the use of the Goldmann one. Place a numbing drop into your patient's eye and place a drop of lubricating solution onto the corneal surface of the lens. Tell the patient to try to keep his lids open and look at your ear while you "use this lens to gently hold his eyelids open." Then, while gently pulling down on the lower lid, place the lens onto the surface of his cornea. Under high magnification, with a bright, narrow slit beam, examine the angle structures. Start with the inferior angle again (the superior mirror), and work your way around alphabetically. When you're done, repeat the process with the other eye.

The Zeiss lens only needs to be applied to the surface of the cornea with minimal pressure. You will know if you are pressing down too hard because you will see folds in the cornea while you're doing your exam. Sometimes, it is actually a beneficial maneuver to press on the cornea while performing gonioscopy with a Zeiss lens. Forbes described a technique where the clinician can press on the cornea to see if a narrow angle can be coaxed into opening[1]. In this procedure, a Zeiss lens is used to observe the angle structures in patients with anatomically narrow angles. As more pressure is applied to the cornea by the lens, aqueous humor is forced out of the center of the anterior chamber and into the angles. Often, by performing this simple technique, deeper aspects of the angle can be seen, and a better estimate of the true occludability of the angle can be made.

RECORDING YOUR FINDINGS

Many systems have been developed to record how the anterior chamber angle structures appear when viewed gonioscopically. They all work on similar concepts. Regardless of which specific system you are taught, you should always record 4 specific bits of information: 1) the depth of the anterior

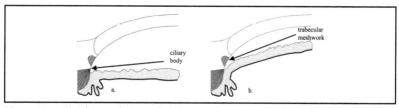

Figure 9-7. (a) This angle is graded 4+ open because everything down to the ciliary body can be seen through gonioscopy. (b) This angle is graded 2+ open because only the trabecular meshwork can be seen.

chamber angle, 2) the angle the iris makes with the cornea, 3) the degree of pigmentation, and 4) the appearance of any abnormalities.

The Depth of the Angle

When examining a patient's angle structures, it is important to comment on whether his angle is "open," "narrow," or "closed." The easiest way to comment on this is to name the most posterior angle structure that can be seen with gonioscopy. If a patient's ciliary body can be seen, his angle is probably wide open, and if only trabecular meshwork can be seen, it is probably fairly narrow (Figure 9-7). Most things in an eye examination are graded on a scale of 1 to 4 (3+ cell, 2+ flare, 1+ corneal guttatae, and so on), and gonioscopy is no different. The trick to making it so easy is that there are four angle structures that you may be able to see. From anterior to posterior, these are Schwalbe's line, trabecular meshwork, scleral spur, and ciliary body. All grading systems are based on which of these structures can be visualized.

One system merely names which structure can be seen. A patient may be described as "scleral spur 360 degrees," while another may be described as "trabecular meshwork superiorly and scleral spur nasally, inferiorly, and temporally." By pressing a narrow angle with a goniolens, you may interpret one patient's angle as "Schwalbe's line 360 degrees, opens to trabecular meshwork with compressive gonioscopy." It is a lot to write, but it does convey the pertinent, useful information.

Another system modifies reporting to the usual 1+ to 4+ system seen elsewhere on your examination. Basically, each structure is assigned to a number value. If Schwalbe's line is the only structure seen, it's a 1+ open angle. If trabecular meshwork is seen, it's 2+ open. If you can see scleral spur, it is 3+ open, and if you can see all the way to ciliary body, it is 4+ open.

Spaeth has come up with a very specific method for describing angle structures.[2] It is an excellent system, however, it is only useful in describing a patient if other clinicians with whom you work are familiar with it. If your clinic uses his system, I suggest you read one of his articles on the subject.

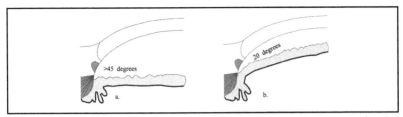

Figure 9-8. (a) This is a grade IV angle because it is greater than 45 degrees. (b) This is a grade II angle because it is only 20 degrees.

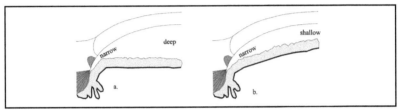

Figure 9-9. (a) At first glance, this patient appears to have a wide open angle because the center of the anterior chamber is deep. Gonioscopic examination, however, reveals "plateau iris," an unusual insertion of the iris root into the ciliary body. In these patients, the chamber angle is actually narrow despite a deep chamber centrally. Compare this patient to one with more typical "narrow angle" glaucoma (b).

The Angle Between the Iris and Cornea

Another indicator of the level of "openness" of a particular patient's anterior chamber angle is the angle the iris makes with the cornea. A normal measure for this is about 45 degrees (Figure 9-8). Larger angles are often seen in pseudophakes and aphakes (because they don't have the crystalline lens pushing the iris forward) and patients with pigment dispersion syndrome. Smaller angles are seen in patients with narrow angle glaucoma or just anatomically narrow angles. In general, an angle that is between 10 and 20 degrees is felt to be occludable, and care should be taken whenever a patient with an occludable angle is dilated.

Some clinicians will describe the iris insertion angle in terms of a grading system. In these cases, a closed angle is grade 0. Grade I is open 10 degrees, Grade II is open 20 degrees, Grade III is between 20 to 45 degrees, and Grade IV is at least 45 degrees. A patient whose angle is open, but is less than 10 degrees, is described as having a "slit" angle.

The specific configuration of how the iris root inserts into the ciliary body is another thing to consider when evaluating the angle. A patient with plateau iris, for example, may have a normal angle between the iris and the cornea, but because of an abnormal insertion of the iris root into the ciliary body, may have structurally narrow angles at the level of the chamber angle

(Figure 9-9). Although most systems of recording findings do not describe this in any great detail, it is usually a worthwhile thing to note, especially in abnormal cases. Spaeth's system uses a "q," "r," "s" system to describe just this.

The Degree of Pigmentation

The next thing to observe and record is the level of pigmentation present in a patient's angle. Most patients will have a symmetric degree of pigmentation when one eye is compared to the other. If one eye has more pigment than the other, it may be a sign of pseudoexfoliation, pigment dispersion, or prior trauma, surgery or inflammation. Level of pigmentation is graded on a scale of 1+ to 4+. The label 4+ pigmentation is usually reserved for patients with a Sampaolesi's line, a line of pigment at the level of Schwalbe's line, seen in patients with pseudoexfoliation or pigment dispersion syndrome. As a general rule, patients with more heavily pigmented angles will respond better to laser trabeculoplasty, so this is an important thing to note.

Abnormal Findings

The last thing to record is the presence of any abnormalities seen during the gonioscopic examination. This group is kind of a *potpourri* of miscellaneous entities, and includes anything unusual that you may see. Included here are angle recession and clefts, tumors and cysts, peripheral anterior synechiae, neovascularization of the angle, and any of a host of things left there after prior surgery (eg, haptics, vitreous, ostea).

REFERENCES

1. Forbes M. Gonioscopy with corneal indentation. A method for distinguishing between appositional closure and synechial closure. *Arch Ophthalmol.* 1966;76:488.
2. Spaeth GL. *Ophthalmic Surgery: Principles and Practice.* 2nd ed. Philadelphia, Pa: WB Saunders;1990.

10

Tonometry

INTRAOCULAR PRESSURE

Years ago, investigators measured the intraocular pressure (IOP) in a large number of people, and found what they felt was a Gaussian curve with a mean of around 16 mmHg (millimeters of mercury). Two standard deviations below the mean was around 10 mmHg, and 2 standard deviations above the mean was around 21.5 mmHg. Based largely on this study, we say that anyone with intraocular pressure greater than 21.5 mmHg has an intraocular pressure that is significantly above that seen in the general population. We label this patient as having *ocular hypertension*, and he runs a risk of developing glaucoma at some point.

It was a good study in a lot of ways because it does give us a number to set as the high normal for IOP. But, it was a flawed study in a lot of ways, also—probably in more ways than it was a good study. First, there was an over-representation of Whites in the patient base, so some experts feel the number 21.5 should be used for Whites, while a different number should be used for other ethnic groups (especially for African Americans whose pressures follow a different curve).

Second, there was an under-representation of elderly in the patient base. As with blood pressures, IOP tends to increase with age. Some investigators feel that the number 21.5 would be too low if a more age-representative patient population were considered. Third, their data did not actually graph out in a true Gaussian distribution, but was skewed toward the higher end. Therefore, the mean/standard deviation calculations that they used to figure out the number 21.5 are not truly accurate. Despite all this, most of us still use the number 21.5 as the upper end of the range of normal pressure.

Patients often confuse high eye pressure with glaucoma. We say, "the pressure in your eyes is a little high today," and they hear, "I have glaucoma."

I will often present the following analogy to help patients understand this difference:

> *High eye pressure is to glaucoma like high blood pressure is to a heart attack. There are many people who spend their whole lives with high blood pressure who never get a heart attack, and there are many who have heart attacks who never had high blood pressure. However, if you do have high blood pressure, your chances of getting a heart attack are higher. The same is true for high eye pressure and glaucoma. If you have high eye pressure, your chances of getting glaucoma over your lifetime are greater than if you don't. However, this doesn't mean that you will automatically get glaucoma, only that your chances are higher.*

This usually helps patients understand the role of high eye pressure in glaucoma.

METHODS OF DETERMINING INTRAOCULAR PRESSURE

The difficult part about measuring a patient's IOP is that you have to measure the pressure *inside* of the eyeball without ever actually putting any instruments in there. We don't have the same luxuries in finding pressure inside of an eyeball as we do in finding pressure inside an airplane cabin or an automobile tire. An airplane cabin is big, and all the people who are directly affected by the pressure are usually positioned within it. Therefore all the pressure sensing and readout devices can be located *inside* the cabin where the pressure needs to be measured.

Techniques to measure the pressure inside an automobile tire must differ from those for airplane cabins for 3 specific reasons. First, the interior of an automobile tire is much smaller than that of an airplane cabin. Second, the interior of an automobile tire is exposed to much more violent movement than that of an airplane cabin (hopefully) making the permanent placement of sensitive pressure measuring equipment impossible. Instead, a pressure-measuring device is applied to the tire only when we wish to know the pressure. Third, while the people who are most interested in the pressure measurements of the airplane cabin are placed within it, those interested in the pressure inside the automobile tire are almost certainly located outside of it. Because of these specific constraints, automobile tire pressure is measured in a much different fashion than airplane cabins.

In a lot of ways, the eyeball is more similar to an automobile tire than an airplane cabin. The eyeball is small, probably wouldn't benefit from permanent placement of a pressure measuring device (although that technology may be here some day for select patients), and the people interested in the measurement are located outside of the eyeball itself (and not within the vitreous or anterior chamber). That, however, is where the similarities between pressure determination in automobile tires and eyeballs end. In measuring tire pressure, we have a decided advantage in that we can actually open up the tire in a controlled way and measure the pressure by directly measuring the air as it tries to escape. We cannot place a valve in the wall of the eyeball to directly measure the intraocular pressure. Methods had to be developed to measure the IOP without actually breaching the protective eye wall.

Fortunately, the material that makes up the eye wall (cornea and sclera) is flexible. If the eye were made of a rigid material like bone, for instance, it would be impossible to determine its IOP without putting the tip of some instrument inside of one of the eye cavities. However, because the eye wall is flexible, we can indirectly measure the pressure inside of the eye by pressing on some part of the eye and observing how it changes shape. Basically, *the greater the force that must be applied to the eye from the outside to get it to change shape, the higher the pressure inside the eye* (the IOP). All commonly used methods of determining IOP depend upon that basic principle. Schiotz tonometry depends upon the theory of indentation, where the *depth* of *indentation* of part of the cornea is measured. Intraocular pressure here can be determined by comparing the depth of indentation to the size of the weight causing the indentation. Other methods of determining IOP (eg, Goldmann applanation tonometry, pneumotonometry) rely on the concept of applanation. With applanation, the cornea is not actually indented, rather, a certain known *area* of cornea is just *flattened* to determine the IOP. Both indentation and applanation tonometry work on the principle that scleral and corneal rigidity is constant from patient to patient.

There is a fairly new wrinkle in this line of thought. For decades, we assumed that intraocular pressure measurement was reasonably consistent from patient to patient because corneoscleral thickness and rigidity were essentially the same among healthy patients. However, studies have shown us that this was not only untrue,[1] but also clinically important.[2] These studies unearthed the observation that patients with thinner corneas had a more progressive glaucoma than patients with thicker corneas despite the fact that their *measured IOPs* were not statistically different. The key to this observation, of course, is that they are talking about the artificial act of measuring the IOP by applanation, and not the true intraocular pressure.

Here is an analogy. Take a balloon, bicycle tire, and automobile tire and fill them up with air so they all have the *same exact pressure*. Now, with your finger, try to determine which one has the highest pressure. The car tire feels firmest because the actual rubber part of the tire wall is thickest, and you will likely be tempted into believing that this one has the highest pressure. Because the wall of the balloon is the thinnest, you will likely be tricked into thinking that this one has the lowest pressure—it just feels softer. Of course, you may believe that the bicycle tire is somewhere in between, but in truth, they all have exactly the same pressure. The lesson here is that when we measure the pressure of something by pressing on it from the outside, we can be fooled.

We can apply this idea to intraocular pressure. Take 3 patients whose true intraocular pressure is 18 mmHg. One has a thin cornea (490 μ), one has an average cornea (540 μ), and one has a thick cornea (590 μ). When we measure their pressures by pressing on the eye with an external measuring device, the thin cornea would measure an incorrect 15 mmHg, the average one would measure 18 mmHg, and the thick one would measure an incorrect 22 mmHg. Let's say that we decide that a pressure of 18 is too high, and we would rather the patient have a pressure of 16. Well, we're mistakenly happy about the thin cornea patient's measurement of 15, so we leave him alone—even though the true pressure is 18. We bring the average patient's IOP down to 16 with one eye drop. The thick patient worries us because of such a high reading (again, even though his true pressure is also really 18), so we put the patient on 2 eye drops to bring the measured pressure down to 16 (bringing the true pressure down to 13 or 14). Because we essentially overtreat our thick cornea patients, we get them into a much safer zone, and they may well do better over time. Because we relax about our thin cornea patients when we should not, they end up being under treated, and can do worse.

Palpation

Every once in a while, you will have a patient that is too young, squeamish, or developmentally delayed to obtain the IOP through any of the techniques described in the following section. In these instances, you can get a general feel of the IOP through palpation as a kind of last resort. To get a palpation IOP, all you need to do is ask the patient to close his eyes, and then just feel his eyeballs with your fingertips through his closed lids. Baum and associates[3] showed that it is very difficult to actually quantitate pressure with a number just by performing palpation. All you should be able to reliably determine is whether the eye feels soft (IOP <6 to 8), hard (IOP >30), or somewhere in between.

Here's a tip. Feel the tip of your nose—the tender part—with your fingertip. If your patient's eye feels like this, it's probably somewhere in the worry-free range (between 6 and 30 mmHg). Now feel your chin (the bony part). If your patient's eye feels like this, his IOP is probably too high. Now feel your cheek. If your patient's eye feels like this, his IOP is probably too low. In my opinion, that's all you need to do. By comparing how your patient's eye feels to different areas of your own face, you should be able to tell whether the intraocular pressure is low, high, or somewhere in between. Then, write in the chart, either: *low to palpation, normal to palpation,* or *high to palpation.*

Schiotz Tonometry

At one time, Schiotz tonometry was the gold standard for measuring a patient's IOP. For various reasons, including inconvenience, difficulty in caring for the equipment, and inaccuracy of readings in certain types of patients, the Schiotz tonometer has pretty well fallen out of favor in eye clin-

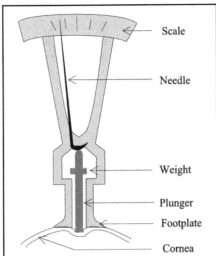

Scale

Needle

Weight

Plunger

Footplate

Cornea

Figure 10-1. The Schiotz tonometer. Note that the plunger indents the cornea, while the footplates, because of their larger surface area, do not. The needle, because it rests on the top of the plunger, records the amount of corneal indentation. This number, which is read from the scale, can be transformed into intraocular pressure in mmHg if the size of the weight is known.

ics. The single basic advantage of the Schiotz tonometer, however, is that it is completely portable. It doesn't rely on any bigger, fancy instruments (like a slit lamp), and it fits snugly in your pocket and does not require access to an electrical outlet. For this reason, it is still fairly widely used in emergency rooms and can still be found in some internist/family practitioner's offices, although even here it is being replaced by the easier-to-use tonopen.

The Schiotz tonometer works on the concept of indentation tonometry (Figure 10-1). The basic idea is that, by applying a weight to the cornea, the eye deforms in such a way that the weight actually *indents* the eyeball. The amount of indentation achieved is a factor of a number of things including corneoscleral rigidity and corneal thickness. However, it is most dependent upon intraocular pressure, the amount of weight applied, and the surface area of the cornea that is being indented. The system is designed so that the amount of applied weight can easily be measured, and the surface area of the indented cornea is constant, meaning that the biggest variable in the equation is the IOP.

Basically, the higher the IOP, the less the globe will be indented by a specific weight. Conversely, the lower the IOP, the more the globe will be indented by that same weight. Schiotz, years ago, used cadaver eyes with known intraocular pressures to experimentally calibrate his tonometer to transform distance of indentation to intraocular pressure when specific weights were applied to a plunger with a known surface area. For the majority of cases, it is very accurate.

The bottom half of the Schiotz tonometer is made up of a footplate and plunger. The footplate, which has a relatively large surface area, rests gently on the cornea. The plunger has a much smaller cross sectional area than the footplate. When a small weight is placed on the plunger, a fairly large pressure (pressure = weight/area) is transmitted through the plunger to the cornea, resulting in a small amount of corneal indentation. The top of the plunger is in contact with a needle that moves in relation to a fixed scale. While the needle can move, the scale is fixed because it is attached to the footplate and not to the plunger. The scale is numbered from 1 to 20, but it is important to realize that these numbers *do not* represent the intraocular pressure. The numbers on the scale are directly related to the distance of indentation, and a conversion table must be used to figure out the intraocular pressure based on the number read off the scale. The size of the weight on the plunger (which can be varied) and the surface area of the end of the plunger (which is constant) are the other factors needed to convert to intraocular pressure in mmHg. Remember that this loses accuracy when measuring pressure in patients with very thick or very thin corneas.

The Schiotz tonometer must be held so that the plunger is perpendicular to the floor, so it is best to use it while your patient is in a supine or near-supine position. First, you must place anesthetic drops into your patient's eye. Next, get everything ready to go—start with the 5.5 g weight on the plunger. After everything is all set, gently hold your patient's eyelids open and place the footplates and plunger of the Schiotz tonometer gently on the cornea. Be sure not to press down on the cornea or eyelids excessively, as this may artificially elevate the IOP. With the tonometer in proper position, merely read the number off the scale to which the needle is pointing. Take the tonometer off the cornea, record the reading, and repeat for the other eye. Once both eyes are done, convert the scale readings to IOP using the table.

Although the scale goes from 0 to 20, it is most accurate from 5 to 15. Therefore, you should use different weights until the scale reads somewhere between 5 and 15 (Table 10-1). For example, let's look at a patient with IOP of 36. With just the 5.5 gram weight on the plunger, the scale reads around 1. This is too low. We replace the 5.5 gram weight with the 7.5 gram one, and the reading on the scale rises to around 3—still too low (we want to be between 5 and 15). We next replace the weight with the 10 gram one, and the scale reads 5.4. Now we can go to the conversion table—look under the 10.0 gram column, to scale reading of 5.4 (5.5 is there), and we read the IOP as about 36 mmHg. It's a lot of work just to get a patient's pressure, and that is why it is not used much any more. However, it is accurate in most situations.

Noncontact Tonometry

Noncontact tonometry is a technique that was developed by Grolman in 1972,[4] as a way to determine a patient's intraocular pressure without actually touching the eyeball. Many patients may remember it as the "eye puff" test. The idea behind noncontact tonometry is that when subjected to a puff of air, the cornea will temporarily flatten. Collimated light is reflected off the cornea, and by evaluating how this light behaves, the amount and nature of the corneal deformation can be recorded. Intraocular pressure can then be

Table 10-1

CALIBRATION CHART FOR SCHIOTZ TONOMETRY[5]

SCALE	WEIGHT ON PLUNGER			
READING	5.5 G	7.5 G	10 G	15 G
0.0	41.4	59.1		
1.0	34.5	49.8	69.3	
2.0	29.0	42.1	59.1	
3.0	24.4	35.8	50.6	81.8
4.0	20.6	30.4	43.4	71.0
5.0	17.3	25.8	37.2	61.8
5.5	15.9	23.8	34.4	57.6
6.0	14.6	21.9	31.8	53.6
6.5	13.4	20.1	29.4	49.9
7.0	12.2	18.5	27.2	46.5
7.5	11.2	17.0	25.1	43.2
8.0	10.2	15.6	23.1	40.2
8.5	9.4	14.3	21.3	38.1
9.0	8.5	13.1	19.6	34.6
10.0	7.1	10.9	16.5	29.6
10.5	6.5	10.0	15.1	27.4
11.0	5.9	9.1	13.8	25.3
11.5	5.3	8.3	12.6	23.3
12.0	4.9	7.5	11.5	21.4
12.5	4.4	6.8	10.5	19.7
13.0	4.0	6.2	9.5	18.1
13.5		5.6	8.6	16.5
14.0		5.0	7.8	15.1
14.5		4.5	7.1	13.7
15.0		4.1	6.4	12.6
16.0			5.2	10.4
17.0			4.2	8.5
18.0				6.9
19.0				5.6
20.0				4.5

ZONE OF GREATEST ACCURACY (spanning scale readings 8.5–15.0)

The diameter of the plunger is constant. If you know the mass of the weight on the plunger, IOP can be determined from the reading off the scale.

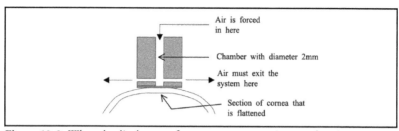

Figure 10-2. When the diaphragm of a pneumotonometer is pressed against a cornea, it decreases the size of the channels through which exiting air must pass, resulting in increased resistance. To overcome this increased resistance, pressure builds in the chamber. When a corneal area with a diameter of exactly 2 mm is flattened by the diaphragm, the pressure within the chamber dips, and, at this point, IOP can be determined.

determined by the nature of the corneal flattening. Noncontact tonometry is not routinely used in the majority of eye clinics, possibly because it is unpopular with patients, and less accurate than tonometry.

Pneumotonometry

Pneumotonometry is the most accurate way of determining intraocular pressure in patients with significant corneal pathology or irregular astigmatism. Pneumotonometers use a probe with a silastic diaphragm covering a chamber with a diameter of 2 mm (Figure 10-2). Air is forced into the chamber in such a way that it must pass between the chamber and the diaphragm before it is allowed to escape. The more external force that is pressed against the diaphragm, the higher the internal pressure must be to overcome the resistance and allow the forced air to escape. This air pressure can be measured as a graph. When exactly 2 mm of the diaphragm is pressed against the flattened cornea, a dip will be seen in the graph, and the difference between the trough of this dip and the baseline of the graph is the IOP.

Pneumotonometers differ from one another based on some of the features that they may offer. Some will print a graph of readings on paper, while others will give a digital readout, for example. For the most part, however, most of the principles behind how different machines work are similar. This type of tonometer works equally well regardless of the position of the patient, so it may be performed in any position the patient finds most comfortable. Because the patient does not need to be supine (as they do for Schiotz tonometry), and do not need to place their head in a slit lamp (like Goldmann applanation tonometry), pneumotonometry is ideal for patients confined to a wheelchair. Also, because readings are equally good whether the cornea or sclera is applanated, it is a good procedure for small children and queasy adults who may perform the Bells phenomenon when you approach with an instrument, and bury their corneas under their upper lids.

To perform pneumotonometry, be sure the patient is comfortably seated. Examine the tip of the tonometer. It should be disinfected between every use according to the policy set up by your clinic. If the tip is wiped with bleach or alcohol, be sure that it is rinsed and dried before touching it to your patient. Be sure a silastic membrane is properly positioned over the tip of the probe. Then, place a drop of anesthetic in your patient's eye and turn on the pneumotonometer, making sure there is good flow of air from the tank through the tip. If the air supply is in any way compromised, most tonometers will give out a warning signal. Gently hold your patient's lids open while asking him to keep both eyes open and look at something across the room. It is important to ask him to look at something far away with the other eye to keep the patient from following the tip of the instrument with both eyes causing him to cross uncomfortably. All that's left to do now is to place the tonometer tip against the patient's cornea (or sclera), and wait for the data to collect. Because you're looking at the patient's eye instead of the machine, most tonometers will let you know when good data has been collected by signaling you with some kind of audible signal (like a "beep"). Record the value and repeat for the other eye.

Tonopen

The tonopen is a handheld electronic instrument that measures intraocular pressure. There are 2 classes of patients in whom the tonopen is the instrument of choice for determining the IOP. The first are those patients with corneal pathology or excessive astigmatism. In these patients, applanation tonometry may be inaccurate, and Schiotz tonometry has other disadvantages as outlined above. The second group is made up of children and patients with developmental delay who may not tolerate applanation or other forms of IOP determination. The mechanism of the tonopen is similar to that of the pneumotonometer, and like the pneumotonometer, the tonopen works equally well on corneas as scleras. For this reason, it is ideal for patients expressing a strong desire to execute the Bell's phenomenon.

Importantly, tonopens must be stored with a rubber sleeve over the tip to avoid damage to the equipment. Whether you store your tonopen with a clean sleeve, ready for the next patient, or a used one from the last patient, will depend upon the policy of your clinic. Policy on how often to calibrate the tonopen also differs from clinic to clinic. When determining IOP via the tonopen, it is important to correctly follow the instructions as outlined by the manufacturer. First, place a drop of local anesthetic into your patient's eyes. Then, holding the instrument like a pen in one hand, gently hold the patient's lids open with your other hand, and ask him to keep both eyes open and focus on something across the room. Be sure that the instrument is on and in the "measure" mode, and tap the tip against the cornea (or sclera) repeatedly until the instrument beeps to let you know it has received an appropriate amount of data. Normally it will average a number of different

Figure 10-3. The Goldmann applanation tonometer is shown pressed against a cornea. When force on the tip flattens an area of cornea with a diameter of 3.06 mm, the intraocular pressure can be read from the dial.

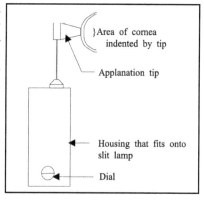

} Area of cornea indented by tip

Applanation tip

Housing that fits onto slit lamp

Dial

readings and give you an accuracy value in addition to the mean IOP value. Record both numbers and repeat the process with the other eye.

Goldmann Applanation Tonometry

Goldmann applanation tonometry is fairly easy to perform because Goldmann has already done all of the hard work. His principle is based on theories of applanation (like in pneumotonometry), where the external force applied to an eye is related to both the intraocular pressure and the area of the cornea being flattened. For pneumotonometry, remember, this area of cornea has a diameter of 2 mm. For Goldmann applanation tonometry, it has a diameter of 3.06 mm.

The precision of Goldmann applanation tonometry depends upon how exactly that 3.06 mm can be measured. This is where the true genius of Goldmann can be realized. He developed a system where the operator can easily examine the flattened area of the cornea and record when it has a diameter of *exactly* 3.06 mm. He developed a biprism that fits onto the slit lamp (Figure 10-3). Anesthetic and fluorescein are placed into the patient's tear film, and the biprism is touched to the patient's cornea while the patient is asked to look at something off to the distance. A meniscus of fluorescein-stained tears forms at the edge of the biprism, and this meniscus can easily be seen when viewed with the blue light of the slit lamp. The biprism splits the image of the meniscus that the clinician sees into 2 semicircles. The clinician can then increase the force of the biprism on the eye by turning the dial at the base of the housing. As the force increases, the flattened area of cornea will grow in size thus changing the size of the 2 semicircles. If not enough force is applied to the surface of the eye, less than 3.06 mm of cornea will be flattened, and the semicircles will be too small and will not overlap (Figure 10-4). If too much force is applied to the surface of the eye, more than 3.06 mm of cornea will be flattened, and the semicircles will be too large and will overlap by too much. If the exact amount of force is applied,

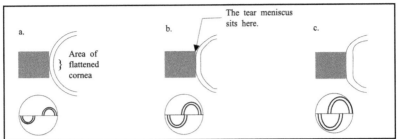

Figure 10-4. (a) The tonometer tip is applied to the cornea with insufficient force. The diameter of the flattened cornea is less than 3.06 mm, and when viewed through the biprism, the semicircles are too small and do not overlap. (b) The tonometer tip is applied to the cornea with the proper force. The diameter of the flattened corneal area is exactly 3.06 mm, and when viewed through the biprism, the inner edges of the semicircles exactly touch. At this stage, the correct IOP can be read off of the dial. (c) The tip is applied to the cornea with too much force. The flattened area is too large, and the semicircles overlap too much.

the area of flattened cornea will have a diameter of exactly 3.06 mm, and the 2 semicircles will be lined up so that the inner edges of the semicircles exactly overlap.

There are a few techniques to learn when performing Goldmann applanation correctly. You will get better results if you use a higher slit lamp magnification and brighter light. Your results may be off if too much or too little fluorescein is used. If the semicircles seem very thick, there is too much dye in the tear film (usually the tonometer tip hit one of the lids), and you should stop and dab the patient's eyelids with a tissue. If the semicircles seem thin and faint, add more dye to the tear film to ensure more accurate readings. If your patient has a lot of astigmatism, the semicircles will actually be semi-ellipses, and this may throw your readings off. If this is the case, measure the pressure with the axis of the tonometer tip in one direction (degrees are printed on the side of the tip), then repeat the reading after you rotate the tip 90 degrees. Then either record both readings or the average of the two. If the patient has a corneal surface that is too irregular, either from trauma, scarring, or prior surgery, the mires may be so irregular that you cannot perform Goldmann applanation tonometry. In these cases, IOP should be determined using pneumotonometry or a tonopen.

Cleaning of the tonometer tips will vary from clinic to clinic. The basic worry is that one tonometer tip is used to touch mucus membranes of different people, and this is potentially a way that viruses can be spread. Some clinics will soak tonometer tips in bleach for 5 to 10 minutes between patients, while others merely wipe them with alcohol. The verdict is still out on what is the best technique. You must bear in mind, though, that both bleach and alcohol will hurt the corneal epithelium. So regardless of which method you use, be sure to rinse and dry the tip off carefully before using it on your patient's eye.

REFERENCES

1. Johnson M, et al. Increased corneal thickness simulating elevated intraocular pressure. *Arch Ophthalmol.* 1978;96:664–665.
2. Medeiros FA, et al. Corneal thickness measurements and frequency doubling technology perimetry abnormalities in ocular hypertensive eyes. *Ophthalmology* 2003;110:1903–1908.
3. Baum J, et al. Assessment of intraocular pressure by palpation. *Am J Ophthalmol.* 1995;119:650–651.
4. Grolman B. A new tonometer system. *Am J Optom & Arch Am Acad Optom.* 1972;49:646.
5. Friedenwald JS. Tonometer calibration. *Trans Am Acad Ophthalmol.* 1957;61:108–123.

11

Ophthalmoscopy

The fundus examination is a difficult skill to learn. First, all the things you need to see are pretty far back there (it's only about an inch, but in the eye, that's pretty far back there). Second, there are often a lot of things between the fundus and your eye that may get in the way of your view. These may include the eyelids, iris, cataract, vitreous debris, or blood—any of which can make your view of the fundus more difficult. Finally, you are essentially looking at a moving target through a keyhole, and the brightness of the light may make it difficult for many patients to keep their eye as still as you may like.

Although a lot of people refer to this part of the examination as the "retina exam," you should get into the habit of calling it the "fundus exam" from the beginning. The basic reason for this is that you are looking at more than just the retina. Do not forget about the vitreous, RPE, choroid, and even the sclera, all of which combine to form the fundus. To call the fundus exam the "retina exam" would be akin to calling the anterior segment exam the "cornea exam." Clearly, there is a lot more to look at than just the cornea.

The first thing you will notice when looking at the fundus is that it is colored kind of an orangey-pinky-yellow, and other than a few blood vessels and a nerve, there are not a lot of obvious landmarks that pop right out at you. The orangey-pinky-yellow color is derived from the combination of all the layers of the fundus. The sclera, way in the back, is white. On top of this is the choroid that is a combination of red blood vessels and brown melanin. In some patients with only a small amount of melanin, these vessels stand out sharply against the white sclera, and in darkly pigmented persons, the melanin may actually make the choroidal vessels difficult to see. In front of the choroid is Bruch's membrane and the single layer of melanin-containing cells known as the retinal pigment epithelium (RPE). While these layers also probably add a little brownness to the whole fundus, unlike the choroid, they are constant from person to person. The retina lies on top of the RPE. The normal retina, remember, is transparent (it has to be because the

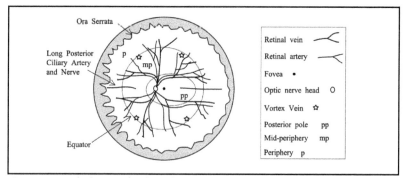

Figure 11-1. The human fundus. The posterior pole, midperiphery, and periphery are separated by dotted lines. Note that the retinal arteries are darker and thicker than nearby retinal veins. Also note that, although arteries may cross veins, arteries never cross other arteries and veins never cross other veins. The 4 vortex veins are deep (at the level of the choroids), and correspond to the anatomic equator.

photoreceptors which react to the incoming light lie way at the back of it), so it doesn't actually add any color to the fundus. The exception to this is in the *macula lutea* (Latin for "yellow spot") where the retina collects a yellow pigment called *xanthophyll*.

GEOGRAPHY OF THE FUNDUS

The fundus can be broken down into a few different geographic zones (Figure 11-1). Starting from the back, the first zone is called the *posterior pole*. This zone, also called the *area centralis* or histologic macula, is where most of the central vision takes place. That means that whatever image you are viewing should fall somewhere in this area. Histologically, the posterior pole corresponds to the area of the retina where the ganglion cells are stacked at least 2 deep. Anatomically, it is the area bordered nasally by the optic nerve head, and superiorly and inferiorly by the vascular arcades. The fovea (or macula lutea) lies in the middle of it.

The most anterior zone is called the *periphery*. The periphery should be thought of as everything from the equator forward. The most anterior aspect of this zone may be quite difficult to see, and require all of your ophthalmoscopic skills. It is an important region to examine, however, because it includes the *ora serrata* and vitreous base, either of which can be responsible for many different types of pathology. The most posterior aspect of the periphery lies at the equator. This region is easy to find in most patients because this is where the internal aspects of the vortex veins lie, and these are quite visible if you know what you're looking for. If you've found the vortex veins, you've found the equator.

Lying between the posterior pole and the periphery is the third region that you need to examine. This region is called the *midperiphery*. It is bor-

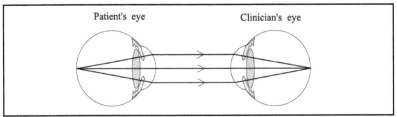

Figure 11-2. Light that starts as a focused point on your patient's fundus will leave his eye as parallel light. Your eye will then focus this parallel light to a point on your fundus.

dered posteriorly by the temporal vascular arcades and anteriorly by the equator. The midperiphery is home to many of the retinal blood vessels. The long posterior ciliary arteries and nerves can also be seen coursing through the midperiphery at the 3- and 9-o'clock positions on their way to the periphery.

METHODS OF PERFORMING A FUNDUS EXAMINATION

The key to examining a patient's fundus lies in managing two specific elements, the optics and the illumination. First let's look at the optics. We have to look at a patient's fundus in such a way that the image of his fundus comes into sharp focus on our own fundus. Only when this happens will we be able to see anything in detail. In a lot of ways, that's trickier than it sounds. After bouncing a light off our patient's fundus, it has to pass through his vitreous, lens, anterior chamber, cornea, and tear film through the air, and then through our tear film, cornea, anterior chamber, lens, and vitreous before hitting our own retina. That is a lot of transparent structures with different refractive indices and curvatures to pass through, but believe it or not, if you are corrected for distance and gaze into the eyes of your emmetropic patient and neither of you accommodates, you should each see the other's fundus in perfect detail (Figure 11-2). The only problem is that the inside of the eye is too dark to make out the details and, therefore, the pupil appears black.

Now, let's look at the illumination. All we need to do is hook up some type of illumination system so that the direction of the incoming light is exactly the same as the direction of our view into the pupil, and the fundus will show up in an orangey-pinky-yellow hue. We are all familiar with this phenomenon from flash photography. Often, when taking pictures of people with a flash camera, the pupils will appear red instead of black. This is due to the camera's flash and lens being located close enough to one another that light from each enters the subject's pupil almost parallel, thus lighting up the inside of his eye in a way that it can be captured on film. If you had powerful enough resolution, you would see that you did not just take a picture of a blurry red pupil, you actually have a detailed picture of your subject's fun-

Table 11.1

OPHTHALMOSCOPIC EXAM TECHNIQUES

METHOD	MAGNIFICATION	-OCULARITY	GEOGRAPHY
Hand-held direct	high (15x)	monocular	posterior
Hruby	high (15x)	binocular	posterior
Noncontact (+60,78,90 D)	medium to high	binocular	posterior/mid
Contact	medium	binocular	posterior
Goldmann	medium	binocular	posterior/mid/periph
Indirect (+14,20,28,30 D)	low (2 to 5x)	binocular	posterior/mid/periph

dus. Professional photographers get around this by separating the flash from the lens. In this way, they are not lighting up the same part of the retina that they are photographing, and the pupil always looks black.

All the different types of ophthalmoscopy differ from one another by those 2 features: optics and illumination. Optically, systems may be either direct or indirect. In direct ophthalmoscopy, you are looking right at your patient's fundus. If you are performing indirect ophthalmoscopy, however, you are not looking right at his fundus, rather, you are looking at a virtual image of the fundus that you have formed by holding up a lens. In terms of illumination, all systems rely on some way of making sure the direction of the light source is the same as your view into your patient's eye (coaxial). Some systems have their own light source while others rely on the slit lamp.

There are many techniques available to perform an ophthalmoscopic exam (Table 11-1). Each has their advantages and disadvantages. In order to be able to properly examine patients presenting with a wide range of pathology, you will need to become proficient in each. What follows is a review of these techniques.

Hand-Held Direct Ophthalmoscopy

Although first described by Purkinje in 1823, von Helmholz was credited for the invention of the direct ophthalmoscope in 1850.[1] If you look at the physics of the direct ophthalmoscope, it may strike you as pretty obvious. The tricky part of the direct ophthalmoscope doesn't lie in the optics; it lies in the illumination. Although not particularly difficult in the 21st century, remember that Purkinje and von Helmholz were doing this before electricity and they had to rely on illumination from candles.

Remember that your emmetropic patient focuses parallel light to a point on his retina (see Figure 11-2). Therefore, any light that starts as a point on the retina will leave the eye as parallel light. Remember that when you are

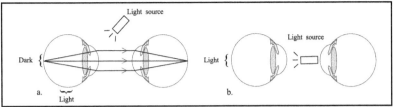

Figure 11-3. A point of light from the patient's fundus emerges from his eye as parallel light and is focused to a point on the fundus of the clinician. In example (a), the light sources comes from above illuminating a peripheral part of the patient's fundus. The posterior fundus is dark because no light is being shone there and the clinician cannot see any fundus details. (b) By positioning the light source between the clinician and the patient, the posterior aspect of the patient's fundus will be illuminated. However, the light source blocks the clinician's view and he cannot see into the patient's eye at all.

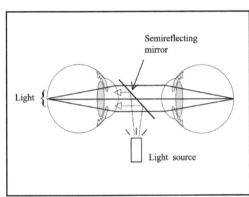

Figure 11-4. The handheld direct ophthalmoscope solves the problems demonstrated in Figure 11-3. The light source is placed below, out of the way of the clinician's view. A mirror is placed in the path of the light source to reflect the light to the posterior part of the patient's fundus. Because the mirror is a semireflecting one, the clinician can see through it to get a view of the patient's fundus.

corrected for distance, you focus parallel light to a point on your retina. It only stands to reason, then, that light that starts as a focused point on your patient's fundus will leave the eye as parallel light that your eye can capture and focus onto a single point onto your own fundus. When that happens, you can see his fundus in perfect detail—assuming you have the proper illumination.

The light must enter your patient's eye in the same direction that you are looking in—it must be coaxial. If it does not, you will end up looking at an area of his fundus that is not illuminated, and everything will look dark (see Figure 11-3). You obviously cannot have the light source placed behind you or your head would block it. Similarly, you cannot have the light source placed in front of you, or it would block your view of your patient's fundus. We get around this problem with mirrors or prisms (Figure 11-4). Most handheld direct ophthalmoscopes are set up with the light source down below in the handle. The light then travels up the shaft until it hits a mirror where it is reflected toward your patient's eye. You look in through a hole in the mirror, so your view in is coaxial to the direction of the reflected light. In this way, you are always sure of seeing an illuminated part of your patient's fundus.

You may notice that your direct ophthalmoscope has a dial on it with black and red numbers. These numbers represent plus (black) and minus (red) lenses built into the head of the ophthalmoscope. These lenses are necessary because you will often be using this instrument to examine patients who are not emmetropic (or you may not be emmetropic and prefer to use it without your glasses on). Because proper functioning of the ophthalmoscope is dependent upon being presented with parallel light, you will need to use these lenses whenever examining an ametrope. If you are examining a myope, remember that light will be exiting his eye in a converging manner, so you will use a minus lens to turn this light into parallel light. If the patient is a −5.00 D myope, you will use the red "5" lens. If you are examining a hyperope, light will be exiting his eye as diverging light, and you'll need to use one of the black lenses to see his fundus in focus. It works out that if you are emmetropic and dial in your patient's refractive error, you should be able to see the fundus in focus. Now let's look at all the techniques available to examine the fundus.

To use the direct ophthalmoscope, have your patient seated comfortably, looking at a specific object across the room. Warn him that you will likely get your head in the way, but he should concentrate on looking to that distant object anyway. If you do not ask the patient to look at a distant target, he will try to look at the ophthalmoscope as you bring it toward him, causing 3 potential problems. First, it will make him cross his eyes, which is uncomfortable. Second, it will place the bright light on the sensitive macula, which can be tough to take. Third, he may try to keep looking at the light source, thus, keeping the macula in your field of view while you are trying to look at other things (like the optic nerve or vessels).

Stand to your patient's side a little bit, turn on the ophthalmoscope and hold it up to your eye. When looking at his right eye, hold the ophthalmoscope in your right hand and look through with your right eye. The scope should be right up against your eye—as close as you can comfortably get it. When looking at his left eye, hold the ophthalmoscope in your left hand and look through with your left eye. It is a lot less clumsy that way, and it will keep you and your patient from bumping noses. Stand about a foot away, close your other eye, and look through the scope with the light on. Turn the lenses until you can clearly see the red reflex through the pupil and note any abnormalities in this reflex (this is similar to the retro-illumination technique described in Chapter 8, and a lot of times, any abnormalities will correspond to cataractous changes of the lens).

Next, open both eyes and concentrate on looking at the red reflex. Move your head slowly toward your patient while keeping his red reflex in sharp focus. Remember to keep the scope up against your eye this whole time. You will probably have to rotate the lens wheel a few clicks to keep things in focus. When the ophthalmoscope is about a half an inch away from your patient's cornea, you should have a view of his fundus. Do not be afraid to get too close. The mistake most new clinicians make is that they end up about 3 or 4 inches away from their patient's eye and stop; this is too far. Think of it as if you're looking at a room through a small keyhole. The closer you can get your eye to that keyhole, the more of the room you're going to see.

The direct ophthalmoscope uses the natural optics of the eye to provide high magnification of fundus structures. Everything seen through the ophthalmoscope will be magnified 15 times. The downside, though, is that you end up with a very small field of view. The field of view with a direct ophthalmoscope is about 3 to 4 disc areas. Because of the high magnification and the small field of view, it is easy to get lost in the fairly featureless expanse of fundus. It is important, then, to find a landmark to figure out exactly where you are whenever performing a fundus examination. The best landmark to find is the optic nerve head because it stands out pretty well against the orangey-pinky-yellow background, and is in just about the same place in everybody.

The optic nerve head is located just nasal to the area of the fundus responsible for central vision (the fovea). Remembering that makes finding it with the direct ophthalmoscope easier; you just have to aim for an area just nasal to his central vision. One way to do this is to have your patient gaze straight ahead while you peek in from the temporal side. That is why it is so important for your patient to look at something located straight across the room while you stand off to his side. If you set everything up just right, the optic nerve head will often be the first thing that pops into view when you do your exam.

Sometimes, however, even though you think everything is set up just right, you will not be looking right at the optic nerve head. When this happens, move the scope around randomly until you find some retinal blood vessels, and follow them one way or the other until they branch. Remember that all retinal blood vessels originate at the optic nerve head, and branch at acute angles. Think of the branching vessels as arrows that point back to the optic nerve (remember back to Figure 11-1). Once you find a vessel, all you need to do is follow it back in the direction the branches point to until you are looking at the nerve.

Once you know where you are, look at the nerve head. Is it a nice healthy pink or is it too red or white? Are the margins sharp or are they blurred? What is the ratio of the cup to the disc? Next follow the vascular arcades in all directions. Note the difference in the caliber of the arteries to that of the veins. Are there any abnormalities where arteries and veins cross? Once you have looked at the vessels in all 4 quadrants, look at the fovea (you can cheat here by asking your patient to look right into the light). Try to find the foveal light reflex. Are there any abnormalities? The high magnification of the hand held direct ophthalmoscope allows for evaluation of even very subtle abnormalities.

Figure 11-5. The Hruby lens is a minus 55 D lens. It takes parallel light leaving the eye, and focuses it as an upright, virtual image located 18 mm behind it. This image is far enough forward that it can be seen in the slit lamp.

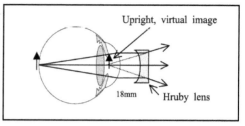

Slit-lamp Ophthalmoscopy With Hruby Lens

The Hruby lens is a lens you can use with the slit lamp biomicroscope to also give you a high-power, low-field view of your patient's fundus. It differs from the hand-held direct ophthalmoscope in 2 specific ways. First, it allows you a binocular view of the fundus, so you can use stereopsis when evaluating fundus structures. Second, it is an indirect method of ophthalmoscopy, which means that you are actually looking at a virtual image of your patient's fundus rather than his true fundus. The Hruby lens is nice for beginners because it has its own slot on most slit lamps—therefore, you do not have to hold it and will not get into any trouble related to a tremor or tilting of the lens.

In an emmetropic eye, remember, light from a point on the fundus emerges as parallel light. A Hruby lens is a −55 D lens that can be placed in front of a patient's cornea, causing this parallel light to diverge (Figure 11-5). A minus lens (covered in Chapter 3) focuses parallel light as a virtual image in negative space. In the case of the Hruby lens, parallel light is focused 18 mm (1/55 D=0.018 meters) behind the lens as an upright, virtual image. The slit lamp can then be used to look at this virtual image, because even though it's a virtual image, you can still see it with the slit lamp—you just cannot project it on a screen.

To use the Hruby lens, position your patient at the slit lamp biomicroscope as you normally do for the anterior segment examination. Set up the light source and the oculars so they are both aimed directly into your patient's eye. Place the Hruby lens into its slot so that the slit beam shines through it and make the slit moderately dim, high, and wide. Set up the fixation light so your patient can easily see it with his other eye while looking straight ahead. Now, just push the oculars forward until the image of the fundus comes into focus. If you have set it all up correctly, and your patient is looking straight ahead, you will probably find yourself looking right at his optic nerve head without even having to move things around too much. It is difficult to move the scope around to view the fundus, but by slowly moving the fixation light in front of the other eye, your patient will move his eye until the proper structures come into view. You can change the magnification by switching the oculars on the slit lamp. When viewing through 16× slit lamp magnification, the magnifica-

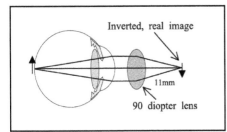

Figure 11-6. The 90 D lens is an example of a high-plus noncontact lens. It takes parallel light leaving the eye and focuses it as an inverted, real image located 11 mm in front of the lens. This image is far enough forward that it can be seen in the slit lamp.

tion will be about equal to that of the hand-held direct ophthalmoscope (about 15x), and the field of view will be about one disc area.

Slit-Lamp Ophthalmoscopy With High-Plus Non-Contact Lens

You can use a high plus lens to view an image of the fundus much the same way you can use a high minus lens (like a Hruby lens). Both lenses focus parallel light to a point somewhere that the slit lamp can view it. While the Hruby lens focuses parallel light to a point in minus space (in the anterior chamber of your patient's eye), the high plus lens focuses it to a point in plus space (between the lens and the slit lamp). While the Hruby lens focuses parallel light to an upright, virtual image, a high plus lens will focus it to an inverted, real image (Figure 11-6).

Different powers of plus lenses can be used with the slit lamp biomicroscope to afford a stereoscopic view of the fundus. The most popular ones are the +60, +78, and +90 D lenses. The +60 D lens gives the greatest magnification while the +90 D lens gives the largest field of view.

To properly use one of these lenses, set the patient up in the slit lamp as if you were doing an anterior segment examination. Align the oculars so you are looking through the pupil along the visual axis. Make the slit a small, dim, rectangle of light, and shine it straight into the pupil in the same direction as the oculars. Be sure not to make the light too bright here—the high plus lens will focus the light to a point that the patient may find uncomfortable. Hold the lens up about 1 or 2 cm in front of your patient's cornea, perpendicular to your slit beam. While looking at his right eye, hold the lens in your left hand, and while looking at his left eye, hold it in your right hand. Hold the lens between your forefinger and thumb and use your other 3 fingers to steady your hand and hold open his lids as needed.

You next have to focus on the real image of the fundus as created by this lens. If you are using a +90 D lens, this image will be 11 mm on your side of the lens (1/90 D = 0.0011 meters), so you will need to pull the oculars of the slit lamp pretty far back in order to see it properly. Look through the oculars of the slit lamp the whole time and watch as your rectangular shaped slit gradually comes into focus. If you have set everything up properly and your patient is looking at your ear with his other eye, you should find yourself looking at his optic nerve. Once things are in focus, you can move the slit around to see the optic nerve head, vessels, and macula. If you want to look at your patient's fovea, merely ask him to look at the small rectangle of light. Remember that, because you are looking at a real image, everything you see will be upside-down and backwards. When you become more adept, you can use this technique to see details in the midperiphery, and with well-dilated, co-operative patients, you can even see some structures in the periphery.

Slit-Lamp Ophthalmoscopy With Contact Lens

For the greatest detailed stereoscopic viewing of the fundus, it is often advantageous to use a contact lens in combination with a slit lamp biomicroscope. Because the contact lens has a flat front surface, and sits on the cornea (thus doing away with the cornea-air interface), it negates the refractive power of the front surface of the cornea. In this way, the optics of the slit lamp can be used to view posterior pole structures with great detail. The contact lens should really be thought of as a Hruby lens that has been pushed so far back that it is actually sitting right on the cornea, and like the Hruby lens, it gives us an upright, virtual image. This type of lens allows us to see the fundus in the greatest detail, probably better than with the high plus noncontact lenses (60, 78, or 90 D), and is best to see subtle findings such as macular edema.

To perform a contact lens fundus examination, place a drop of topical anesthetic onto your patient's eye. Next, put some type of lubricating liquid onto the surface of the lens that is to go against your patient's cornea. This liquid will help couple the lens to the cornea and decrease refractive aberration as the light passes from the lens to the cornea. If you think your patient may need funduscopic photographs taken after you see him, I recommend that you don't use anything too thick here (anything greater than 2.5% carboxymethylcellulose), because it will make the tear/air interface irregular and cause the pictures to come out blurry. With the patient positioned at the slit lamp, gently pull down the lower lid and place the bottom part of the lens into the cul-de-sac. Then ask him to look up, and slip the upper part of the lens under the upper lid margin. Next ask him to look at your ear or the fixation light with his other eye and aim the slit through the pupil until you see a red reflex. Slowly push the oculars of the slit lamp forward until the red-reflex becomes focused as a rectangle of sharply focused fundus. If you have set everything up properly and the patient is looking at your ear, you will likely be looking right at his optic nerve head.

Using this type of contact lens will allow you to examine the posterior pole with fairly high magnification, and excellent detail. However, as with direct ophthalmoscopy, you do sacrifice field of view. It is difficult to see different areas of your patient's posterior pole by moving the slit beam around

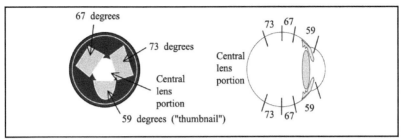

Figure 11-7. The Goldmann 3-mirror lens is really 4 lenses in one. The clear central portion allows you to see the posterior pole. The 73-degree mirror allows you to see the midperiphery, and the 67- and 59-degree mirrors allow you to see the periphery. The 59-degree mirror can also be used to view the anterior chamber angle structures.

and tilting the lens. The easiest way to expand your view is to move the fixation light and have your patient move his eye for you. In this way, you should be able to visualize a large amount of the posterior pole with minimal discomfort to the patient.

Slit-Lamp Ophthalmoscopy With Goldmann 3-Mirror Lens

The Goldmann 3-mirror lens is really 4 lenses in a single carrier. The central part functions like the contact lens described above, and is superb for viewing the posterior pole under medium to high magnification. Around this central lens are 3 mirrors, each at a different angle, which together allow for high magnification viewing of the entire fundus (Figure 11-7).

To correctly use this lens, sit the patient comfortably at the slit lamp and place a drop of topical anesthetic into his eye. Place a thick lubricating drop onto the surface of the lens that is to go against the cornea and have him look at a fixation light with the other eye. While telling the patient that you will be using a special lens that will hold the eyelids open, put the bottom of the lens against his lower lid margin, ask him to look up, and place the top of the lens under the upper lid margin. This is a big lens, so you may need to get the lids open wide in order to fit it in there. Aim a dim rectangular beam through the middle of the lens, and move the oculars forward until it comes into focus. To get a good view of the posterior pole, merely move the fixation light around while reminding your patient to look at it.

The steepest mirror is angled at 73 degrees and allows you to see the midperiphery. To use this mirror, move the slit beam from the center of the lens over to the mirror. Move the oculars until the slit beam is in focus on the fundus. Remember that this is a flat mirror, so the image you are seeing is an inverse one of the fundus located 180 degrees away. The mirror has a fairly small field of view, but by tipping the lens a little one way and the other, you should be able to increase the amount of fundus you can see through it. Once you've examined a particular area of the midperiphery, merely rotate the lens to bring another area into view. By rotating the lens a full 360 degrees, you should be able to visualize the entire midperiphery. Remember that this is a big lens and it doesn't have a flange to help you keep it in place. You need to be careful as you rotate it and tip it, or the patient may squeeze it out during your manipulations.

To see a band of fundus that is more anterior, switch to the next mirror. This mirror is angled at 67 degrees and will allow you to examine the anterior aspect of the midperiphery and the posterior aspect of the periphery. This mirror should be used in the same manner as the previous one, remembering, again, that the image in the mirror is an inverse one of the fundus located 180 degrees away. Once the fundus is examined with the second mirror, move the slit so you are looking through the third one. This third mirror is angled at 59 degrees and is shaped like a thumbnail. It is probably most commonly used as a goniomirror when the patient is undilated (see Chapter 9), but it can also be used to see the far periphery when your patient is fully dilated.

By using all 4 parts of the Goldmann 3-mirror lens, you can actually see the entire fundus. However, the high magnification and the small fields of view make this an inefficient lens to use in this manner. If you use this lens alone, you are likely to miss a lot of important bits of pathology. The Goldmann 3-mirror lens is best used to get a closer look at a specific area that you've localized through some other method (such as indirect ophthalmoscopy).

Indirect Ophthalmoscopy

The indirect ophthalmoscope is probably one of the hardest things to learn how to use in the eye clinic, one of the few things that is harder than gonioscopy. Not only do you have to somehow coordinate the position and movement of both of your hands, your head, your eyes, and your patient's eyes, but you then have to process the fact that the image that you see in the lens is backwards and upside-down.

The biggest advantage to indirect ophthalmoscopy is that it provides a look at the fundus with a large field of view. Remember that most of the other techniques described above may provide a field of view measuring anywhere from 1 to 10 disc areas in size. With indirect ophthalmoscopy, you should be able to see an area 1 to 2 times the size of the whole posterior pole in one view. The other advantage to indirect ophthalmoscopy is that it allows you to see far out in the periphery with minimal effort and manipulation.

There are 2 basic disadvantages to using the indirect ophthalmoscope. The first is that the magnification is quite low. This is a trade-off, of course, for the large field of view, but is does take practice to make out a lot of detail

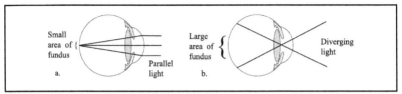

Figure 11-8. (a) Light from a small, focused area of fundus will leave the eye as parallel light. (b) Light from a larger area of fundus will leave the eye as diverging light.

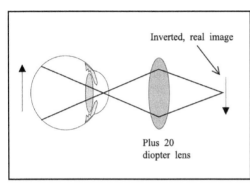

Inverted, real image

Plus 20
diopter lens

Figure 11-9. The condensing lens takes the diverging light that leaves the eye and focuses it to an inverted image in real space. The clinician can then see this image with an indirect ophthalmoscope. Although the image is located between the condensing lens and the ophthalmoscope, to the clinician, it will appear to be within the lens.

using this technique. The second disadvantage is that, because you are actually looking at a real image of the fundus created by the plus lens, everything you see in the lens will be upside-down and backwards and this can be confusing when you're just getting started. If you remember, the high-plus noncontact lenses will give a similar inversion when used with a slit lamp biomicroscope (see above).

It is important to understand what makes it the indirect ophthalmoscope different than the other types of ophthalmoscopy described above. All the other forms of ophthalmoscopy work on the principle of taking *parallel* light leaving your patient's eye and focusing it onto your own fundus. They all process parallel light because of the idea that light that leaves the eye as parallel light must have started as a focused point on the fundus. This idea is great for seeing detail, as described above, but, unfortunately, this is also where the limitation to field of view comes in. All parallel light that leaves the eye is going to be limited in size by the pupil—you just can't get the image from a large area of fundus to leave the eye as parallel light because the iris is always going to block a large part of it (Figure 11-8).

However, you can get the image from a large area of fundus to leave the eye as *diverging* light. The trick just comes in developing a way of capturing and using all of that diverging light. Indirect ophthalmoscopy has been developed to do just that (Figure 11-9). With indirect ophthalmoscopy you place a high plus (+14, 20, 28, or 30 D) lens between your patient's eye and the indirect ophthalmoscope. This lens takes light that leaves your patient's eye in a diverging nature, and *condenses* it so that it will fit into your own pupil. Most textbooks will refer to the lens as a *condensing* lens.

The condensing lens takes the light emerging from your patient's eye and focuses it as a real image in plus space (somewhere between the lens and your eye). You then have to look through the indirect ophthalmoscope, which you wear on your head, and bring that image into focus on your own fundus. Because it is a real image, and it is located less than 20 feet away from your eye, you will actually have to accommodate to see it clearly. Of course, the more you lean in, moving your head closer to the image, the more you will have to accommodate to see it. Therefore, unlike direct ophthalmoscopy where it is best to move your eye as close to your patient's as you can, in indirect ophthalmoscopy, it is best to stay as far away as comfortable. Arm's length is usually the best working distance here. There are other, optical, reasons why it's best to stay at arm's reach, but that is beyond the scope of this discussion. (If you are interested, I recommend you read Colenbrander's chapter on the subject in Duane's.[1])

Your field of view will change somewhat depending on the condensing lens you choose. The standard lens most of us use is the 20 D double aspheric lens. This provides a 3× magnification. The 30 D lens will provide a relatively larger field of view, but only provides 2× magnification. The 14 D lens provides a relatively smaller field of view with 5× magnification. In a strange twist of physics, you will actually get more magnification and a smaller field with a lower power lens (eg, 14, 20 D) than you will with a higher power one (28, 30 D). This is because you are using the lens as a condensing lens, and not a magnifying lens. For this reason, the lower power lenses are used when you want better magnification, while the higher power lenses are used when you want a larger field of view, or are examining smaller eyes, or through smaller pupils. The 28 D and 30 D lenses are the standard when examining small children and infants.

Because indirect ophthalmoscopy is so difficult but so important, it is helpful if you get yourself in the habit of doing it the same way every time. At some point in your career, you are going to come across difficult situations. It may be that the patient is uncooperative; it may be that you know there is pathology in there, but you just can't find it. In either case, if you have done your exam the same way consistently every time, there will be just that much less you have to think about during these tough exams.

With that in mind, the first thing I recommend you always do when performing indirect ophthalmoscopy is to do it with the patient lying back. Although indirect ophthalmoscopy can be performed with the patient sitting up, you should get in the habit of lying the patient back when performing it. Always make sure that the room is set up in such a way that there will be room for you to walk around at the top of your patient's head when he is lying back. You will be spending a fair amount of your time walking around up there during the indirect ophthalmoscopy exam.

Place the indirect ophthalmoscope on your head and adjust the buckle in the back so the fit is snug but not tight. Turn on the light and look through the eyepieces of the ophthalmoscope. Make sure the interpupillary distance is set for you appropriately. Next, make sure the light source is pointing in the right direction. Hold your hand out at arm's length with the palm facing you. Adjust the light so that it hits your palm when your hand is held in the superior half of the field of the scope. Warn your patient that the light is very bright, but that you will not be using it for a very long time (and try to keep your promise).

The condensing lenses that you use are not spherical; they are aspheric—not only that, but they are double aspheric (meaning that each surface is aspheric). This is important in ensuring that the image is clear all the way out to the periphery. Double aspheric lenses are not symmetric. If you're not careful, you may hold it upside-down which will give you a distorted image. Most double aspheric lenses have a white ring built into the plastic rim on one side. This white rim is fit into the bottom side of the rim. If you hold the lens so that the white rim faces your patient, you are holding it correctly.

Always examine your patients' eyes in the same pattern. I recommend that you always examine the right eye first and examine all the clock hours in a clockwise fashion. When that eye is done, examine the left eye in a counter-clockwise fashion. Resist the temptation to examine the left eye first when that is where the patient's complaints are. You may forget to examine the right eye after finding something interesting in the left.

Hold the lens off to the side, and move your head so that you see a red reflex in your patient's pupil through the ophthalmoscope. Next, hold up the condensing lens between your patient's eye and yours (with the white ring toward your patient) in the path of the light from the scope. While getting started, intentionally hold the lens so it's too close to you—about 8 inches away from the patient is a good distance. By doing this, you should be able to see a nice red reflex in the condensing lens. Now slowly move the lens in toward your patient's eye, all the time keeping the red reflex centered in the lens. It sounds simple, but this is the tricky part because the image is inverted. When you get to the right distance away from your patient's eye, you should see an image of his fundus suddenly fill the whole lens. At this point, you will find it useful to rest your third, fourth, and fifth fingers on your patient's cheek or forehead to steady your hand. I will often use my third finger to hold open his lid if I need to.

You should divide your patient's eyes into quadrants (in your mind), and examine them quadrant-by-quadrant. It is often uncomfortably bright for the patient when you're looking at the posterior pole, so I recommend you save that part of the examination for the end. It is best to start off with the periphery and midperiphery. While you are examining a specific quadrant, you should ask them to look in that direction. For example, if you are trying to examine the superotemporal quadrant of the right eye, ask the patient to look up and to the right. Some patients seem to get the hang of this easily, while others may not. For these patients, it is helpful to remind them to keep both eyes open. Many have the inclination to squeeze closed the eye you are not examining, thus burying the other eye (the one you're interested in) under their brow via the bell's phenomenon. If this does not take care of the problem, have the patient hold out one thumb, and you position it where you want the patient to look (this looks better when asking the patient to look down). Then all you have to say is, "look at your thumb." Most patients can manage this—even in a dark room.

Lay the patient back and stand by his right shoulder. As you examine the different quadrants of his retina, you will effectively be walking around his head. Start by examining the 12-o'clock position in the right eye with the condensing lens in your right hand. Then look from 12 o'clock to 3 o'clock in a clockwise fashion. When you get to the 3-o'clock position, put the lens in your left hand and examine the eye from the 3- to 6-o'clock positions. By the time you're done here, you should find yourself near the top of your patient's head, but still on his right side. Now, step around so you're standing toward the top of your patient's head by the left ear. Hold the lens in your right hand, and examine (still in a clockwise fashion) from 6 o'clock to 9 o'clock. Finally, switch the lens to your left hand and examine from 9 o'clock back to 12 o'clock. You should finish up next to the patient's left shoulder.

Next, you will examine the left eye in a similar fashion—only counter-clockwise this time. You're already standing by your patient's left ear, so you will hold the lens in your left hand to look from 12 o'clock to 9 o'clock; then hold the lens in your right hand to look from 9:00 to 6:00. Next, step around to the other side of your patient's head, put the lens back in your left hand, and look from 6 o'clock to 3 o'clock. Then put it back in your right hand to finish up from 3 o'clock to 12 o'clock. At this point, you have walked around your patient's head again, and should find yourself near his right shoulder—right where you started.

Once you have had a good look at the periphery and midperiphery, you should evaluate the posterior pole. Don't tell the patient to look right into the light—it is very bright. Rather, hold your free hand out in front of him and say, "look at my hand." If you hold your hand in the right place, you'll almost always have his optic nerve centered in your condensing lens when things are in focus.

Scleral Depression

There are 2 reasons why we have to learn to perform a good scleral depressed exam. First, at some point in your career, you will have to find some pathology in the retina that is anterior to the equator (see Figure 11-1). The only way to see things way out there is to deform the eye in such a way that is visible through the pupil. The scleral depressor is the instrument that does this deforming.

Second, because the scleral depressor is not held still, it is slid back and forth along the eye in an antero-posterior direction, it will give us clues to the 3-D nature of what we are looking at. If we just look at something without scleral depressing, we can see that something is there. However, we may not be able to tell if it is depressed, flat, or raised. If you remember, we came across a similar problem when performing a slit lamp examination (see Figure 8-2). We were lucky here because what we were interested in evaluating was so far anterior that we could change the direction of the slit beam to give us clues.

However, because retinal pathology is so far posterior, we cannot use that technique here. Instead, we use scleral depression. By rubbing the tip of the scleral depressor back and forth along the eye, we impart some motion on the part of the eye that we are trying to examine. Raised things will appear different when in motion than depressed things, and so on. Flap tears may even seem to wave at you as the depressor distorts the eye beneath it.

When first learning to handle the scleral depressor, just use it to gently hold the lid; do not try to do any real depressing. This will get you into the habit of using it without causing discomfort to the patient. Try not to press on the tarsus of the lid, as this can be uncomfortable—even with minimal pressure. Aim for the creases. Make sure that the tip of the depressor is at least 1 cm above the lid margin of the upper lid, and a 0.50 cm below the margin for the lower one.

The hardest part comes next—you have to make sure that everything lines up. There are three things that always have to be in a straight line: 1) the ophthalmoscope, 2) the scleral depressor, and 3) the condensing lens. If they don't line up exactly, you probably won't be able to see what you're trying to see. It is easiest to line up your ophthalmoscope with the scleral depressor without the lens there, so hold the lens away from the pupil to get started. Once the scleral depressor is lined up with the ophthalmoscope, slip the lens into place, and everything should look the way it is supposed to. If things get out of line, remove the lens and get the depressor lined up with the ophthalmoscope. Do not try to line things up with the lens in the way because it creates an upside-down image, and this makes things more difficult.

Then, once everything is lined up properly, you should gently run the depressor over the eyelid in a front-to-back motion. This step should be gentle, and the patient should not experience discomfort. If the patient complains, you are probably pressing too hard. After you have looked at 1 clock hour to your satisfaction, move to the next in the order described above keeping all 3 points (ophthalmoscope, lens, depressor) in a perfect line. If you lose the image, take away the lens, line things up, then return the lens. After you have done 3 clock hours, you should switch which hands you are holding the lens and depressor in, and continue on.

Once the right eye is complete, do the left eye in the same fashion. Only this time, you'll be examining the eye in a counter-clockwise fashion. When you see something, comment to yourself the clock hour where it is and move on. This is the easiest way for you to remember it.

You do not typically need to put in any numbing eye drops when performing a scleral depressed exam; remember, if a patient complains, you are probably doing it too hard. However, there is 1 exception to this rule. If you really need to take a close look at the 3- and 9-o'clock areas (eg, for new floaters), it may be difficult to do a scleral depressed exam here because the lids do not cover these areas well. In these instances, it may be beneficial to put in some numbing drops, warn the patient that *things may feel funny here for a few minutes*, then put the depressor directly on the sclera. If you warn the patient and are gentle, you can almost always do this without undue trauma or anxiety.

Some practitioners are wary of starting right in using a metal scleral depressor and may wish instead to use something softer like a cotton-tipped applicator. Because the average cotton-tipped applicator is bigger than the average scleral depressor, you may end up struggling more to get it in the proper position, and may cause the patient more discomfort that you would with a metal scleral depressor. I recommend that you get in the habit of starting out with a metal depressor from the get-go. After all, they are designed to do that job.

RECORDING WHAT YOU SEE

Different methods exist for recording findings from a fundus examination. Some methods rely on writing out what is seen, while others rely on drawing pictures. Either method is adequate when done properly, although most agree that specific pathology should probably be drawn. As we discussed for the anterior segment examination, a standardized system has been established for color-coding fundus pathology. It is summarized in Table 11-2.

Every time you perform a fundus examination, be sure to comment on the view in, optic nerve, vessels, macula, and periphery.

View In

The "view in" is a very important part of the fundus examination, and probably the one most forgotten. The basic idea behind recording the view in is that if a patient's retina, visual pathways and brain are all normal, your view in should be equal to his visual acuity. If, because of cataract or corneal scarring for example, you can only see his retina with 20/50 sharpness and his visual acuity is 20/50, you can assume that his anterior segment pathology is probably causing most of his decreased visual acuity. However, if you have a patient with 20/70 visual acuity and a 20/20 view in to his retina, you need to take a close look at his fundus. If his fundus looks normal to you, this patient may need to have further testing done (eg, visual field, contrast sensitivity, VEP, MRI).

Table 11.2

SYSTEM FOR DRAWING THE FUNDUS EXAM

COLOR	PATHOLOGY
Red	Attached retina, retinal hemorrhage
Blue	Detached retina, vessels
Brown	Pigment
Yellow	Lipid exudates
Green	Anything obscuring your view (cataract, vitreous hemorrhage)
Orange	Infiltrate, drusen

Optic Nerve

The next thing to look at is the optic nerve. When performing most kinds of ophthalmoscopy, this should be the first thing you find because it gives you a landmark and lets you know exactly where in your patient's fundus you are. The first observation to make about an optic nerve is its color. A normal optic nerve is pink because it is made up of fairly equal parts of red (blood vessels) and white (nerves and supporting glia). An abnormal nerve may appear too red or too white. If it appears too red, it is usually because there is too much blood. Flame hemorrhages or capillary congestion from papilledema are two examples of times when the nerve may appear too red. If it appears too white, it is usually because there is too much glia or too little blood. Optic atrophy and myelinated nerve fibers are 2 good examples of this.

The second feature of the optic nerve to evaluate is the margin. The margin of the optic nerve that you can see is actually made up of Bruch's membrane, the choroid, and the sclera—structures that underlie the nerve fiber layer of the retina. Because the retina and nerve fiber layer are normally transparent, these margin structures can clearly be seen and a normal nerve has a margin that can be described as *sharp*. However, if the nerve fiber layer swells (as in papilledema), it will lose its transparency and your view of the underlying structures will become less sharp. When this happens, the disc margin can be described as *blurred*.

The last feature to describe about the optic nerve head is the cup to disc ratio. What this describes is how much of the optic nerve head is actually taken up by nerve fibers, and is most important in describing patients with glaucoma. Almost all patients have dimples in their optic nerve heads to some degree or another. This dimple is labeled the *cup* because it represents a hollow structure of a certain volume (like a drinking cup). The optic nerve head itself is referred to as the *disc* because it is flat and, from the front, looks like a disc (Figure 11-10). It is made up of all the nerve fibers coursing their way back to the brain from the retina. You need to record how big the

Figure 11-10. Three different optic nerve heads are shown from the top (above) and the side (below): (a) shows a cup to disc ratio (c:d) of 0.10 meaning that the cup takes up only 10% of the area of the disc; (b) shows a c:d ratio of 0.50; and (c) shows a c:d of 0.95.

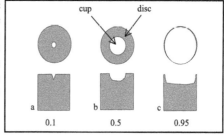

cup is in relation to the disc, and there are a number of different ways that you can do this.

One system describes the ratio of the size of the cup to the size of the disc (the cup-to-disc ratio, or cup:disc, or c:d). It's nice that you only have to think of it as a ratio between the two because that way you don't have to know their actual sizes. You just have to know the relationship of one to the other. The cup to disc ratio will always be somewhere between 0.0 and 1.0 (it only goes up to 1.0 because the cup can never be bigger than the disc). If the cup is really small compared to the disc, the c:d will be small (0.1 or 0.2). If the cup is really large compared to the disc, the c:d will be large (like 0.8 or 0.9).

Another system will look at the linear ratio in both the horizontal and vertical directions. In this system, you may record 0.5 horizontal and 0.6 vertical. Some practitioners will go a step farther and divide each line in half. They may record that the ratio of cup-to-disc is 0.2 inferiorly, 0.3 nasally, 0.4 superiorly, and 0.4 temporally. Remember here that each ratio is on a scale from 0.0 to 0.5 because we're only looking at half of each line.

Regardless of how you define the nerve mathematically, it is important to draw what the nerve looks like too. Different patients with the same c:d may have completely different looking optic nerve heads. Only by drawing it can you show specific areas of nerve tissue thinning, sloping, or frank loss. This is especially important when dealing with patients with glaucoma who may have very focal, but sight-threatening, areas of disc margin thinning or notching. In the clinic, you will likely supplement your drawings with more technologically advanced forms of data analysis such as photography, ocular coherence tomography, or nerve fiber analysis.

Vessels

The fundus is one of the only places in the body where arteries and veins are laid out for all to see. This is a very important concept to understand. If a diabetic has a lot of damage to the vessels in his fundus, the chances are good that there is also damage to the vessels of his kidneys, heart, and brain. The same goes for the hypertensive patient. Therefore, by carefully examining our patients' vessels when performing a fundus examination, we can help in the management of systemic disease.

Although the retinal, choroidal, vortex, and ciliary vessels are all visible during fundus examination, the retinal vessels are the ones that give us the most information about systemic disease. The retinal arteries and veins enter the eye at the optic nerve head and branch out to cover almost the entire fundus (the fovea is notably spared). When looking at the retinal vessels, what you are actually looking at is the column of blood within the vessel lumens. The vessel walls, themselves, are invisible to fundus examination.

The retinal veins, with their deoxygenated blood, appear darker than the retinal arteries. In addition, the retinal veins appear fatter than the nearby retinal arteries—the ratio of the caliber of a retinal vein to that of a nearby retinal artery is usually about 3:2 to 4:3. This is so because the arteries, which represent a high pressure system, have thicker walls and smaller lumens than the retinal veins. Because we are only seeing the lumens and not the vessel walls, the veins appear larger. In certain disease states, most notably hypertension, the artery walls may become abnormally thickened thus making the arterial lumens smaller. When this is the case, the vein to artery ratio may increase to 2:1 or 3:1, a finding that should make the clinician suspicious of atherosclerotic or hypertensive vasculopathy.

Diabetics may present with many different types of vascular abnormalities, but it is beyond the scope of this text to summarize them here.

Macula

The macula is the area of the fundus where the central visual image is projected. The retinal vessels tend to course *around* the macula in a relationship that helps maximize visual acuity (it is difficult to see through blood). Because of xanthophyll pigment, the macula has a yellowish look to it. Sitting in the middle of the macula is a depression called the *fovea*. When your microscope light hits the fovea properly, you will see a reflection that has been labeled the *foveal light reflex*. This is an important clue to be able to recognize because it may be the first thing to disappear in cases of subtle retinal pathology.

Any and all abnormalities of the macula must be described. Abnormalities will include things that are degenerative (drusen), inflammatory (posterior uveitis), structural (macular hole), neoplastic (melanoma), traumatic (chorioretinal scar), vasculopathic (sub-retinal neovascular membrane), infectious (toxoplasmosis), and congenital (Best's vitelliform dystrophy).

Periphery

The last part of the fundus examination to report on is the periphery. Structurally, the periphery is an important area to look at. First, because it is where the retina is thinnest, it is the area most likely to develop small holes or tears. Second, it is where the vitreous and retina are most firmly attached.

Changes in the adherent vitreous can cause pulling of the thin retina causing a retinal tear or even detachment. High myopes are especially at risk because they may have a normal amount of retina stretched thin to cover their longer than average eyes. These thin areas combined with potentially abnormal vitreous will make them much more likely to have a retinal detachment than the rest of the population.

The best way to visualize the periphery is through indirect ophthalmoscopy, especially in combination with scleral depression. The Goldmann 3-mirror lens may also be used, but because of the high magnification and the small field of view, this technique is best used to get a higher magnification view of an abnormality that has already been found with indirect ophthalmoscopy. As with the macular examination, all abnormalities must be recorded.

REFERENCES

1. Colenbrander A. Principles of Ophthalmoscopy. In Duane TD, Jaeger EA (eds): *Clinical Ophthalmology*. Vol 1. Harper & Row, Philadelphia, 1985.

APPENDIX A

Common Abbreviations

A

ABMD	Anterior basement membrane dystrophy
A/C	Anterior chamber
ACL	Anterior chamber lens
AFx	Air fluid exchange
AIDS	Acquired immunodeficiency syndrome
AK	Astigmatic keratotomy
ANA	Antinuclear antibody
ARMD	Age related macular degeneration
AVx	Anterior vitrectomy

B

BC	Base curve
BDR	Baseline diabetic retinopathy
BID	Twice a day
BSCL	Bandage soft contact lens

C

CA	Corneal abrasion
CAI	Carbonic anhydrase inhibitor
CB	Ciliary body
CC	Chief complaint
CC	With correction

CCAG	Chronic closed angle glaucoma
c:d	Cup to disc ratio
CL	Contact lens
CME	Cystoid macular edema
CMV	Cytomegalovirus
CN	Cranial nerve
CNVM	Choroidal neovascular membrane
CPEO	Chronic progressive external ophthalmoplegia
CR	Cycloplegic refraction
C/S	Contrast sensitivity
C/S	Cortical spoking
CSA	Cyclosporine A
CSME	Clinically significant macular edema
CT	Computerized tomography
Ctx	Contacts
CU	Corneal ulcer
CVF	Confrontation visual field

D

DM	Diabetes mellitus
D&Q	Deep and quiet
DR	Diabetic retinopathy
DVD	Dissociated vertical deviation

E

EBV	Epstein-Barr virus
ECCE	Extracapsular cataract extraction
ED	Epithelial defect
EKC	Epidemic keratoconjunctivitis
EOG	Electro-oculogram
ERG	Electroretinogram
ERM	Epiretinal membrane
ESR	Erythrocyte sedimentation rate
ET	Esotropia

F

FA	Fluorescein angiogram
FB	Foreign body
FHx	Family history
5-FU	5-fluorouracil

G

gt	Drop
gtt	Drops
GVF	Goldmann visual field

H

HCL	Hard contact lens
HPI	History of present illness
HSV	Herpes simplex virus
HT	Hypertropia
HVF	Humphrey visual field

I

ICCE	Intracapsular cataract extraction
ICG	Indocyanine green
ID	Identification
INO	Internuclear ophthalmoplegia
IO	Inferior oblique
IOFB	Intraocular foreign body
IOL	Intraocular lens

IOOA	Inferior oblique overaction
IOP	Intraocular pressure
IPD	Interpupillary distance

J

J	Jaeger
JXG	Juvenile xanthogranuloma

K

KP	Keratic precipitate
KPE	Kelman Phacoemulsification

L

LASEK	Laser assisted sub-epithelial keratomileusis
LASIK	Laser assisted in situ keratomileusis
LH	Lid hygeine
LK	Lamellar keratoplasty
LLL	Left lower lid
LR	Lateral rectus
LUL	Left upper lid

M

MDF	Map-dot-fingerprint dystrophy
ME	Microcystic edema
MGD	Meibomian gland dysfunction
MMC	Mitomycin C
MP	Membrane peel
MR	Medial rectus
MR	Manifest refraction
MRI	Magnetic resonance imaging

N

NKDA	No known drug allergies
NPA	Near point of accommodation

NPC	Near point of convergence
NPDR	Nonproliferative diabetic retinopathy
NS	Nuclear sclerosis
NV	Neovascularization
NVD	Neovascularization of the disc
NVE	Neovascularization elsewhere

O

OD	Right eye
OHTN	Ocular hypertension
ON	Optic nerve
OS	Left eye
OU	Both eyes

P

PCL	Posterior chamber lens
PCO	Posterior capsular opacification
PDR	Proliferative diabetic retinopathy
PEK	Punctate epithelial keratopathy
PG	Present glasses
PI	Peripheral iridodotomy
PK	Penetrating keratoplasty (also PKP)
PMHx	Past medical history
POAG	Primary open angle glaucoma
POHx	Past ocular history
PPDR	Preproliferative diabetic retinopathy
PPV	Pars plana vitrectomy
PRK	Photorefractive keratectomy
PRN	As needed
PRP	Panretinal photocoagulation

PSC	Posterior subcapsular cataract
PTK	Phototherapeutic keratectomy
PVD	Posterior vitreous detachment
PVR	Proliferative vitreoretinopathy
PXF	Pseudoexfoliation

Q

QD	Every day
QID	Four times a day
QOD	Every other day

R

RAPD	Relative afferent pupillary defect
RD	Retinal detachment
RF	Rheumatoid factor
RGP	Rigid gas permeable contact lens
RK	Radial keratotomy
RLL	Right lower lid
RP	Retinitis pigmentosa
ROP	Retinopathy of prematurity
RUL	Right upper lid

S

SC	Without correction
SCL	Soft contact lens
SL	Suture lysis
SO	Superior oblique
SoHx	Social history
s/p	Status post
SPCIOL	Sutured posterior chamber IOL
SR	Superior rectus
SR	Suture removal
SRNVM	Subretinal neovascular membrane

T

Th	Thickening
TID	Three times a day
TID	Iris transillumination defect
TM	Trabecular meshwork

U

URI	Upper respiratory infection

V

Va	Visual acuity
VH	Vitreous hemorrhage

VKH	Vogt-Koyanagi-Harada syndrome
VZV	Varicella-zoster virus

W

WsP	White without pressure

X

XT	Exotropia

Y

YAG	Neodymium: yttrium-aluminum-garnet laser

Z

APPENDIX B

Common Surgical Procedures

CORNEA

Penetrating Keratoplasty (PK, PKP)

A round, full thickness excision of diseased cornea is performed, and a donor corneal button is sewn into its place. This procedure is also called a corneal transplant.

Lamellar Keratoplasty (LK)

The anterior, diseased part of a cornea is removed, and a donor corneal button is sewn into its place. The patient's endothelium and posterior stroma are left in place.

Superficial Keratectomy

The superficial diseased surface of the cornea is removed. The epithelium is normally allowed to merely grow over the surgical bed. The majority of the patient's corneal thickness is left in place.

Triple Procedure

A combination of three procedures—penetrating keratoplasty, removal of cataract, and placement of an intraocular lens implant.

REFRACTIVE PROCEDURES

Radial Keratotomy (RK)

Radial, near full-thickness incisions are made in the cornea to flatten it, thus making the patient less myopic.

Astigmatic Keratotomy (AK), Limbal Relaxing Incision (LRI)

Near full-thickness incisions are made in the cornea parallel to the limbus to reduce astigmatism.

Photorefractive Keratectomy (PRK)

The epithelium is removed. The excimer laser is then used to reshape the front surface of the corneal stroma to alleviate refractive errors. The epithelium then grows back over 2 to 4 days.

Laser Assisted in Situ Keratomileusis (LASIK)

An anterior corneal flap is made with an automated microkeratome, and the surgical bed is reshaped with the excimer laser to alleviate the refractive error. The corneal flap is laid back down, and stays in place without suturing.

Laser Assisted Sub-Epithelial Keratomileusis (LASEK), Epi-LASIK

The corneal epithelium is removed as a single sheet either chemically (LASEK) or mechanically (epi-LASIK). The corneal stroma is then reshaped with the excimer laser to alleviate the refractive error. The epithelium is then replaced where it stays in place without suturing.

Phakic Intraocular Lens Implant (Phakic IOL)

A lens implant is placed in the eye to alleviate refractive errors, without removal of the crystalline lens. The lens implant can be placed in the posterior chamber or the anterior chamber.

Refractive Lens Exchange (RLE)

The noncataractous crystalline lens is removed, and an intraocular lens implant is placed, to alleviate high refractive errors. Technically, this surgery is identical to cataract removal with intraocular lens implantation.

Conductive Keratoplasty (CK), Laser Thermal Keratoplasty (LTK)

Concentric circles of burns are made in the mid-peripheral cornea using radio energy (CK) or laser (LTK). The scarring causes central steepening of the cornea, thus correcting hyperopia.

Intracorneal Ring Segments

Plastic ring segments are placed circumferentially in the mid-peripheral corneal stroma to flatten the cornea to treat low levels of myopia.

GLAUCOMA

Trabeculectomy

A low resistance, partial thickness pathway is made from the anterior chamber to the sub-conjunctival space in order to decrease intraocular pressure.

Trabeculotomy

Usually only beneficial for certain types of congenital glaucoma, an instrument or suture is passed inside Schlemm's Canal for three to twelve clock hours, and manipulated so that the medial wall of the canal is broken allowing aqueous access to Schlemm's Canal with less resistance.

Tube Shunt, Seton

A tube is placed into the anterior chamber, and connected to a plate which is sutured to the sclera under the conjunctiva, allowing the aqueous humor to bypass poorly functioning trabecular meshwork. This device may be necessary for patients with multiple prior surgeries, because the scarred conjunctiva will increase the chances that a trabeculectomy will fail.

Goniotomy

Usually only beneficial for certain types of congenital glaucoma, a knife is passed across the anterior chamber, anterior and parallel to the iris, to open up the anterior chamber angle structures on the opposite side.

Peripheral Iridotomy (PI) or Peripheral Iridectomy (PI)

Once a surgical procedure, this is normally performed with the nd:YAG laser for the treatment of angle closure or narrow angle glaucoma. A hole is made in the peripheral iris to allow access of aqueous humor from the posterior to the anterior chambers. A surgical PI may also be made as part of other surgical procedures such as trabeculectomy, or cataract extraction with intraocular lens implantation.

Argon Laser Trabeculoplasty (ALT), Selective Laser Trabeculoplasty (SLT)

A laser is used with a mirrored lens to make small burns in the anterior trabecular meshwork. When the burns heal, they cause scarring and restructuring of the trabecular beams which result in a decrease in resistance to aqueous flow and subsequent decrease in intraocular pressure. SLT is more selective for pigmented tissue, and causes less histologic evidence of tissue damage than ALT.

CATARACT AND INTRAOCULAR LENS

Phacoemulsification (KPE)

The nucleus and epinucleus of the cataract are removed by phacoemulsification (ultrasound), usually through a small incision. The cortex is removed by irrigation and aspiration. The posterior capsule, zonules and lens fornices are left in place to support the intraocular lens implant. Because phacoemulsification is normally performed through incisions ranging in size from 2 to 3 millimeters, final incision size is determined by the size and type of lens implant that is to be put in.

Extracapsular Cataract Extraction (ECCE)

The nucleus and epinucleus are removed together, in one piece, via expression. The cortex is removed by irrigation and aspiration. The posterior capsule, zonules and lens fornices are left in place to support the intraocular lens implant. An eleven millimeter incision is normally needed to deliver the lens nucleus in one piece.

Intracapsular Cataract Extraction (ICCE)

The entire lens, including nucleus, cortex, capsule, and zonules, are delivered in an *en bloc* fashion. A 180 degree limbal incision is needed to facilitate this type of cataract removal. No capsular support is left for placement of an intraocular lens implant.

YAG Capsulotomy

A neodymium:YAG laser is used to make an opening in the opacified posterior capsule that may form months to years after otherwise successful cataract surgery.

Secondary IOL

Placement of an intraocular lens in a patient who had previous cataract extraction without intraocular lens placement. This lens may be a posterior chamber IOL, and anterior chamber IOL, or it may be sutured to the sclera or iris.

Intraocular Lens Exchange

An intraocular lens is removed, and a different intraocular lens is placed. The new lens may be a posterior chamber IOL, an anterior chamber IOL, or may be sutured to either the sclera or iris.

Combined Procedure

Removal of the cataract (usually via phacoemulsification) and implantation of an intraocular lens implant combined with trabeculectomy.

RETINA AND VITREOUS

Anterior Vitrectomy (AVx)

Anterior vitrectomy is normally performed during anterior segment surgery, where anterior vitreous is removed from an incision anterior to the pars plana. No attempt is made to remove posterior vitreous. Vitreous may be removed either by engaging it with a cellulose sponge and cutting with scissors, or by introducing the automated vitrector with or without a light pipe. Another name for anterior vitrectomy is subtotal vitrectomy.

Pars Plana Vitrectomy (PPV)

Three stab-incisions are made through the pars plana. An irrigating port, light pipe, and automatic vitrector are inserted to remove as much of the vitreous as possible.

Scleral Buckle (SB)

For years the standard of care for the treatment of retinal detachments. During a straightforward buckle, the interior of the eye is not entered, and the retina is not directly handled. Instead, a plastic surgical element is wrapped around the eye to change its shape and relieve the internal forces (usually vitreous) acting to cause the detachment. Scleral buckling is normally done in combination with cryotherapy or laser.

Pneumatic Retinopexy

Often small detachments caused by retinal holes can be managed without scleral buckling or pars plana vitrectomy. Air or gas is injected into the eye to lay the detached retina flat and prevent more fluid from gaining access to the subretinal space.

Panretinal Photocoagulation (PRP)

PRP is the standard of care in the treatment of proliferative disease of the retina be it from diabetes, arterial occlusion or sickle-cell anemia. The idea is that peripheral retinal tissue is ischemic because of poor circulation, and secretes a factor into the vitreous that causes new vessel formation. Unfortunately, these new vessels normally cause a lot more harm (traction retinal detachments, vitreous hemorrhages) than good. Therefore, treatment is aimed at their resolution. PRP entails selective ablation of the ischemic peripheral retinal tissue with laser, to stop the source of the new vessel growth factors.

Focal Macular Photocoagulation

Some disorders of the retina (diabetes, vein occlusions) will result in the collection of fluid within the macula causing a decrease in visual acuity. Often, leaking microaneurysms can be sealed with laser burns. If specific areas of leakage cannot be seen, the sub-retinal structures can be irritated with laser causing them to take up the extra fluid. In either case, the burns are of much smaller duration, diameter and power than burns used in panretinal photocoagulation.

Other disorders of the retina (macular degeneration) will cause formation of abnormal blood vessels under the retina. These can be destroyed using a different form of focal laser treatment.

Photodynamic Therapy (PDT)

Abnormal sub-retinal blood vessels are activated with intravenous injection of a medical dye, then ablated using a low level laser. This is similar to focal ablation, but gentler because only the abnormal vessels retain the dye and thus are destroyed by the laser.

STRABISMUS

Resection (Rs)

An extraocular muscle is removed from the globe, a distal segment of it is removed, and the remaining muscle is sewn back to its original place. This acts to shorten a muscle and move the eye toward the operated upon muscle.

Recession (Rc)

An extraocular muscle is removed from the globe and sewn back into place farther back from the limbus. This acts to, in effect, lengthen a muscle and move the eye away from the operated upon muscle.

Transposition (Tp)

All or part of one or more than one muscle is moved to perform the function of a neighboring paralytic muscle.

PLASTIC AND RECONSTRUCTIVE

Ptosis Repair

The eyelid of a patient with ptosis is lifted so that the lid margin sits higher.

Pseudoptosis Repair or Blepharoplasty

The anterior lamella of an eyelid (skin, orbicularis muscle), and often prolapsed orbital fat are removed in a patient with dermatochalasis (also known as pseudoptosis). The lid margin height is not altered.

Dacryocystorhinostomy (DCR)

An opening is made connecting the floor of the nasolacrimal sac to the anterior nasopharynx to treat patients with obstruction of the nasolacrimal system at the level of the nasolacrimal sac or below.

Tarsal Strip

The lower lid is tightened by reattaching the lateral aspect of it to the periosteum of the lateral orbital wall. This is used for patients with problems related to lower lid laxity.

APPENDIX C

Dosages of Common Medication

DILATING DROPS

Sympathomimetic Mydriatics

Hydroxyamphetamine hydrobromide 1%
Phenylephrine hydrochloride 2.5%, 10%

Cycloplegics

Atropine sulfate 0.5%, 1%, 2%, 3%
Cyclopentolate hydrochloride 0.5%, 1%, 2%
Homatropine hydrobromide 2%, 5%
Scopolamine hydrobromide 0.25%
Tropicamide 0.5%, 1%

ANTIBIOTICS

Commercially Available Antibacterial Solutions

Chloramphenicol 0.5%
Ciprofloxacin (Ciloxan) 0.3%
Gatifloxacin (Zymar) 0.3%
Gentamicin sulfate 0.3%
Levofloxacin (Quixin) 0.5%
Moxifloxacin (Vigamox) 0.5%
Ofloxacin (Ocuflox) 0.3%
Sulfacetamide sodium 10%, 15%, 30%
Sulfasoxazole diolamine 4%
Tobramycin sulfate 0.3%
Polymyxin B/Neomycin .... 3.5 mg/ml

Polymyxin B/Neomycin/Gramicidin .... 0.025 mg/ml
Polymyxin B/Trimethoprim (Polytrim) .... 1 mg/ml

Commercially Available Antibacterial Ointments

Bacitracin zinc .... 500 u/g
Chloramphenicol 1%
Erythromycin 0.5%
Gentamicin sulfate.. 0.3%
Sulfacetamide sodium.. 10%
Sulfisoxazole diolamine 4%
Tobramicin 0.3%
Polymyxin B/Bacitracin .... 500 u/g
Polymyxin B/Neomycin .... 3.5 mg/g
Polymyxin B/Neomycin/Bacitracin .... 400 u/g
Polymyxin B/Oxytetracycline.. 5 mg/g

Fortified Antibiotic Solutions

Bacitracin .... 9600 units/ml
Cefazolin .... 54 mg/ml
Gentamicin.. 14 mg/ml
Penicillin G... 333,000 u/ml
Tobramycin... 15 mg/ml
Vancomycin... 33 mg/ml, 50 mg/ml

Injection Dosages of Common Antibiotic Agents

Medication	Sub-Con-Junctival	Intra-Vitreal	Intravenous
Amikacin	25 mg	0.4 mg	15 mg/g/d/3 doses
Ampicillin	50 to 150 mg	0.5 mg	4 to 12 g/d/4 doses
Bacitracin	5000 units	--	--
Carbenicillin	100 mg	0.25 to 2 mg	8 to 24 g/d/4 to 6 doses
Cefazolin	100 mg	2.25 mg	2 to 4 g/d/3 to 4 doses
Ceftazidime	200 mg	2.20 mg	1 g/d/2 to 3 doses
Clindamycin	15 to 50 mg	1 mg	1 to 1.8 g/d/2 to 3 doses
Colistimethate	15 to 25 mg	0.1 mg	2.5 to 5 mg/kg/d/2 to 4 doses
Erythromycin	100 mg	0.5 mg	--
Gentamicin	10 to 20 mg	0.1 to 0.2 mg	3 to 5 mg/kg/d/2 to 3 doses
Kanamycin	30 mg	--	--
Methicillin	50 to 100 mg	1 to 2 mg	6 to 10 g/d/4 doses
Neomycin	125 to 250 mg	--	--

Penicillin G	0.5 to 1 mil u	--	12 to 24 mil u/d/4 to 6 doses
Polymixin B	10000 u	--	--
Ticarcillin	100 mg	--	200 to 300 mg/kg/d
Tobramycin	10 to 20 mg	0.1 to 0.2 mg	3 to 5 mg/kg/d/2 to 3 doses
Vancomycin	25 mg	1 mg	15 to 30 mg/kg/d/ 2 to 3 doses

Topical Antifungal Medications

Amphotericin B .... 0.1 to 0.5%
Flucytosine 1%
Natamycin 5%
Miconazole 1%

Topical Antiviral Medications

Idoxuridine (IDU) 0.1%
Trifluridine (Viroptic) 1%
Vidarabine (Vira-A ointment) 3%

ANTIBIOTIC STEROID COMBINATIONS

Combination Antibiotic and Corticosteroid

Blephamide ointment (sulfacetamide-prednisolone)
FML-S suspension (sulfacetamide-fluoromethalone)
Neodecadron solution (neomycin–dexamethasone)
Poly-Pred suspension (neomycin-polymyxin B-prednisolone)
Pred-G suspension (gentamycin-prednisolone)
Pred-G ointment (gentamycin-prednisolone)
TobraDex suspension (tobramycin-dexamethason)
TobraDex ointment (tobramycin-dexamethasone)

ANTI-INFLAMMATORIES

Topical Corticosteroids

Dexamethasone solution (Decadron) 0.1%
Dexamethasone ointment (Decadron) 0.05%
Dexamethasone sodium phosphate solution 0.1%
Fluorometholone ointment 0.1%

Fluorometholone suspension 0.1%, 0.25%
Fluorometholone acetate suspension...0.1%
Loteprednol solution (Alrex, Lotemax) 0.2%, 0.5%
Prednisolone acetate suspension 0.12%, 0.125%, 1%
Prednisolone sodium phosphate solution..................................0.125%, 1%
Rimexolone 1%

Topical Nonsteroidal Anti-Inflammatory Drugs

Bromfenac (Xibrom)... 0.1%
Diclofenac (Voltaren)... 0.1%
Flurbiprofen (Ocufen) 0.03%
Ketorolac (Acular) 0.5%
Nepafenac (Nevanc) 0.1%
Suprofen (Profenal)... 1%

Topical Anti-Allergy Medications

Azelastine (Optivar)... 0.05%
Epinastine (Elestat)... 0.05%
Ketotifen (Zaditor) 0.025%
Levocabastine (Livostin).. 0.05%
Olopatadine (Patanol) 0.1%
Pemirolast (Alamast) 0.1%

Anti-Glaucoma Medications

Direct-Acting Cholinergic Agents

Carbachol..0.75%, 1.5%, 2.25%, 3%
Pilocarpine 0.25%, 0.5%, 1–5%, 6%, 8%, 10%

Indirect-Acting Cholinergic Agents

Demecarium 0.25%, 0.5%
Echothiophate 0.03%, 0.06%, 0.125%, 0.25%
Physostigmine.. 0.25%, 0.5%

Sympathomimetics

Dipivefrin hydrochloride..0.1%
Epinephrine bitartrate... 2%
Epinephrine borate 0.5%, 1%, 2%
Epinephrine hydrochloride...0.5%, 1%, 2%

Beta-Blockers

Betaxolol (Betoptic) 0.25%, 0.5%
Carteolol (Ocupress) 1%
Levobunolol (Betagan) 0.25%, 0.5%
Metipranolol (Optipranolol) 0.3%
Timolol (Timoptic, Betimol, Istalol) 0.25%, 0.5%

Hyperosmotics

Glycerin (Osmoglyn) .... 50% ....1 to 1.5 g/kg ....oral
Isosorbide (Ismotic) .... 45% ....1.5 g/kg ....oral
Mannitol (Osmitrol) ....5 to 20% .... 0.5 to 2 g/kg IV
Urea (Ureaphil)....................... 30% .... 0.5 to 2 g/kg IV

Oral Carbonic Anhydrase Inhibitors

Acetazolamide (Diamox) .... 125, 250, 500 mg
Dichlorphenamide (Daranide) .... 50 mg
Methazolamide (Glauctabs, MZM, Neptazane) .... 25, 50 mg

Topical Carbonic Anhydrase Inhibitors

Dorzolamide (Trusopt) 2%

Alpha-2 Agonists

Brominidine (Alphagan) 0.15%, 0.2%

Prostaglandins

Bimatoprost (Lumigan) 0.03%
Latanoprost (Xalatan) 0.005%
Travoprost (Travatan) 0.004%

Topical Carbonic Anhydrase Inhibitors

Dorzolamide/timolol (Cosopt)

Eye History and Physical Exam Pocket Guide

EYE HISTORY

ID: Name, age, race

Chief Complaint (cc):
What brought the patient in to see you

History of Present Illness (HPI):
In chronological order

Past Ocular History (POHx):
Don't forget eyeglasses and contact lenses

Past Medical History (PMH):
Especially HTN, diabetes, thyroid

Review of Systems (ROS):

Medications:
Don't forget eyedrops and over-the-counters

Allergies: And what the allergic reaction was

Family History (FHx): Ask specific questions

Social History (SoHx):
Including vocation, avocations and habits

---

copy and clip

EYE PHYSICAL

Visual Acuities (Va):
   Without glasses (sc) at 20 feet
   With current glasses (cc) at 20 feet
   With pinhole (ph) at 20 feet
   With current glasses at 14 inches
Manifest Refraction (MR): Distance and near
Motilities and Alignment:
Confrontation Visual Fields (CVF):
Color Vision:
Pupils: (Shape, size, speed of reaction, ?RAPD)
External Examination:
Slit Lamp Examination:
   Lids/lashes/adnexa (L/L/A)
   Conjunctiva and sclera (C/S)
   Cornea (K)
   Anterior chamber (A/C)
   Iris (I)
   Lens (L)
   Anterior vitreous (V)
Intraocular Pressures: (Methods used and time)
Gonioscopy:
Dilating Drops: (Which drops and time)
Fundus Examination: (Don't forget the view in)
   Macula (M)
   Periphery (P)
   Vessels (V)
   Optic nerves (color, margins, cup:disc)

copy and clip

Index